CREATING THE HOSPITAL GROUP PRACTICE

CREATING
THE HOSPITAL
GROUP
PRACTICE

The Advantages of Employing
or Affiliating with Physicians

ERIC LISTER AND TODD SAGIN

ACHE Management Series

Your board, staff, or clients may also benefit from this book's insight. For more information on quantity discounts, contact the Health Administration Press Marketing Manager at (312) 424-9470.

13 12 11   5 4 3 2

Lister, Eric, 1948-
   Creating the hospital group practice: the advantages of employing or affiliating with physicians/ Eric Lister and Todd Sagin.
      p. ; cm.
   Includes bibliographical references and index.
   ISBN-13: 978-1-56793-330-7 (alk. paper)
   ISBN-10: 1-56793-330-0 (alk. paper)
   1. Hospital-physician relations. 2. Group medical practice. I. Sagin, Todd. II. Title.
   [DNLM: 1. Hospital Administration. 2. Group Practice—organization & administration. 3. Hospital-Physician Relations. WX 150 L773c 2009]
   RA971.9.L57 2009
   362.17'2—dc22

                                    2009020840

Found an error or typo? We want to know! Please email it to hap1@ache.org, and put "Book Error" in the subject line.

For photocopying and copyright information, please contact Copyright Clearance Center at www.copyright.com or (978) 750-8400.

Project manager: Jennifer Seibert; Acquisitions editor: Eileen Lynch; Cover designer: Anne LoCascio

Health Administration Press
A division of the Foundation of the
American College of Healthcare Executives
One North Franklin Street
Suite 1700
Chicago, IL 60606
(312) 424-2800

We would like to dedicate this book to our families, whose love and support make our work possible.

We would also like to thank all of the many hospital and health system leaders whom we have worked with during our years in healthcare. It is these interactions with creative and caring board members, administrators, and physicians that have informed our insights and made our careers so satisfying and productive.

Contents

Preface

THE RESULTS OF NUMEROUS STUDIES evaluating the adequacy of
healthcare in America have been discouraging. Surveys by the
Commonwealth Fund and others show the country trails significantly behind its westernized peers despite a much higher resource
expenditure.[1] Don Berwick and colleagues (2008) have argued that
improving the U.S. health system "requires simultaneous pursuit of
three aims: improving the experience of care, improving the health
of populations, and reducing per capita costs of health care." To
accomplish this triple aim, we must develop new models of care
delivery that powerfully integrate critical resources.

In a health system resistant to comprehensive change, successful
reorganization is not likely to result from a widely accepted, top-
down master plan. In some areas, however, care delivery is under-
going rapid and pervasive revision from the ground up. The advent
of hospitalists is one example of rapid change unmediated by policy or regulatory drivers. The trend central to this book—increasing hospital employment of physicians—is another example.

We are convinced that the increased employment of physicians
is here to stay and that it will come to define medical practice in the
United States—even in the few states that prohibit hospitals from
directly employing doctors.[2] The implications of this change are profound for hospital and health system leaders, patients, policymakers,

and physicians. We believe that powerful multispecialty group practices tightly aligned with hospitals and health systems will emerge and improve both care delivery and resource utilization. As a result, they will set the bar for high-performing health systems of the future. While the Commonwealth Fund and others have touted integrated care as essential to improvement, "nominal" integration is meaningless. Only deeply rooted, broad integration will make the necessary difference. We also believe these groups will place physicians in key leadership roles as prime drivers of health system decision making.

For some, this trend may seem like a déjà vu. The wave of physician employment in the late 1980s and early 1990s fizzled out ignominiously. Hospitals took huge losses and wound up divesting the practices they had purchased at a dear price only a few years earlier. These are different times, however, and the players have learned from past mistakes.

In this book, we have three goals.

The first is to make sense of the movement toward physician employment and to explain why we are convinced that the trend is a fundamental shift and will not reverse again.

The second goal is to cull lessons from the first wave of physician employment and translate them into a road map to success.

The third goal, and perhaps most important, is to propose that there is not just a semantic distinction but a crucial difference between owning disaggregated physician practices and creating a partnership with an employed group practice. We will argue that only the latter model is a sustainable and effective strategy. In making this case, we will lay out what we see as the group practice advantage, as well as the complex, daunting, but ultimately rewarding path to group creation.

Critical questions confronted us as we developed this argument:

- Generational differences affect commitment to work/life balance, attitudes toward practice, and comfort with technology. Given these differences, how do we accommodate both younger and older physicians?

- In designing an employment strategy, how does a hospital relate to physicians who wish to remain in traditional practice settings? How are rivalries dampened, collaboration enhanced, and seamlessness ensured? When is competition between employed physicians and independents appropriate, and when is it disastrous?
- If organizing into a group practice requires some sacrifice by the entity as a whole, what must individuals give up, and how does an organization engender the willingness to do so?
- How do we untangle the Gordian knot of fair compensation? What do we reward? How should we measure productivity? How do we acknowledge indirect contributions to health system success?
- How is the migration to employment changing physicians' attitudes about practice? What is being lost? Is it threatening or possibly destroying time-honored definitions of professionalism?

By addressing these and other questions, we hope to not only explain the advantage conferred by organizing practitioners into groups but honestly confront the dilemmas involved. We will move beyond a theoretical frame of reference by providing concrete guidance to hospital executives and physician leaders who are embarking on the challenge of group creation.

Only in tightly aligned partnerships between physicians and hospitals—the institutions that provide care for our sickest patients—can we hope to deliver truly integrated care. Only truly integrated care will meet the expectations of our patients, provide a rewarding work environment for professionals, constrain healthcare costs while satisfying payers' demands for value, and meet the calls for greater quality and safety sounding loudly from every quarter. Quoting Berwick and colleagues (2008) again, "The pain of the transition state—the disruption of institutions, forms, habits, beliefs, and income streams in the status quo—is what denies us, so far, the enormous gains on components of the Triple Aim that integrated care could offer."

We have written this book to provide guidance through that transition state. As we elaborate in the pages that follow, we are convinced that health systems tightly aligned with well-integrated multispecialty group practices are the most promising vehicle for delivering the future we all seek in healthcare.

Eric Lister, MD
Todd Sagin, MD, JD

NOTES

1. Studies by the Commonwealth Fund can be found on its website at www.commonwealthfund.org.

2. These prohibitions are discussed in Chapter 12. In every state there are alternative vehicles for physician employment that make the arguments of this book germane even to these jurisdictions.

How to Use This Book

IN THIS BOOK, we make a case for the organization of hospital-employed physicians into effective, integrated multispecialty group practices. We bridge theory and practice to explain and clarify our recommendations and offer guidance. Because readers will have varying familiarity with the issues presented, we have divided the book into four parts. Those conversant with the dynamic marketplace changes driving physician employment can start with Part II. If the reader is thoroughly familiar with the subject of multispecialty group practice, Part III may be the most relevant place to begin.

Part I (chapters 1–4) begins with a historical summary of changes in the workforce and in the practice of medicine to set the stage for our discussion of hospital–physician relationships. We proceed by identifying the forces driving physician employment (Chapter 3) and the skills required to develop an effective employed physician workforce (Chapter 4). Readers versed in these issues can skip to Chapter 5.

Part II (chapters 5–9) takes us into the heart of our thesis. We describe the difference between straightforward physician employment and the organization of employed physicians into a group practice, and then map the journey to group practice formation. Chapters 7–9 detail the governance, leadership, and cultural elements that underpin successful groups.

Part III (chapters 10–12) provides critical detail about what must happen within a hospital's group practice to achieve and sustain an advantage in quality, service, and operational efficiency. We focus on the infrastructure of the group practice, operational issues, and legalities. Further, we distinguish between the group practice and the hospital medical staff and describe how reassignment of traditional medical staff duties to the group practice can promote implementation of higher standards.

In Part IV (chapter 13 and conclusion), we show how committed, high-functioning groups can provide their parent health systems with leadership and strategic advantage in the marketplace. In conclusion, we propose that group-led healthcare systems are best positioned to provide the seamless, integrated care demanded by today's discerning consumers.

PART I

CHAPTER 1

The Changing Nature of Hospital–Physician Relations

WHILE THE MAJORITY OF THIS BOOK is designed to provide guidance for the future, there is value to beginning with a lightning-fast overview of modern medicine in the United States. Many of today's issues concerning hospitals and their physicians are rooted in the last century and need to be understood to make sense of current struggles and appreciate the forces and values that will impinge on any change initiative.

THE EVOLUTION OF HOSPITAL–PHYSICIAN RELATIONSHIPS THROUGH THE TWENTIETH CENTURY

Doctors and hospitals have always needed one another, especially since the early twentieth century, when the chances of benefitting from a hospital stay rose above the breakeven point. As the sophistication and efficacy of hospitals grew, they became essential workshops for physicians. The hospital became the most visible symbol of the dramatic scientific advances of twentieth-century medicine, and physicians enjoyed the prestige that accompanied affiliation with a reputable institution. In 1916 the influential American College of Surgeons advocated a selection process to ensure that only qualified doctors were admitted to the staffs of U.S. hospitals.[1]

In 1919 this same group, driven by concerns over quality and a desire to support hospitals committed to professional standards, instituted a formal requirement that hospitals seeking its approval organize the physicians affiliated with them into a "definite medical staff." Organized medical staffs as we know them today were developed as a result, designed to help doctors and hospitals meet common quality goals. In later years, government regulatory bodies cemented this arrangement by requiring that every hospital participating in federal insurance programs have an organized medical staff.[2]

For much of the early twentieth century, physicians were intimately involved in the management of hospitals and, in some cases, were outright owners of these facilities. Financially, the interests of doctors and hospitals were aligned, and what satisfied the needs of one generally satisfied the needs of the other. When the Great Depression threatened the economic well-being of healthcare providers, two companies—Blue Cross and Blue Shield—were created to ensure cash flow to hospitals and doctors. The expansion of federal health programs in the 1960s (Medicare and Medicaid) offered doctors and hospitals retrospective, cost-based reimbursement. Both hospitals and physician practices thrived under this payment arrangement. For the most part, incentives were aligned.

The explosion of medical specialties after World War II anchored the position of the hospital as the center of the medical practice community. The rapid development of expensive medical technologies required that new cohorts of specialized physicians spend most of their time close to their new tools. Cost-based reimbursement supported long hospital lengths of stay, and most physicians had large numbers of hospitalized patients to attend. The professional lives of most doctors were spent in hospitals or nearby offices.

A strong sense of professional community was fostered as a result, and with it physicians developed a feeling of loyalty to their "medical home." In general, hospital medical staffs were open to all applicants as long as they met minimum quality criteria. Growth in the number of medical school graduates in the 1960s and 1970s prompted expansion of hospital medical staffs. A community physician without at least one hospital affiliation was a rarity, and membership on multiple medical staffs became more common.

The growing complexity of hospitals not only required physician staffing in a range of specialties but also a new breed of healthcare administrator better prepared to manage the expanding and more complex institutional bureaucracies. Initially, hospital administrators simply served the physicians working in their facilities. The postwar economic expansion and excellent reimbursement climate of those times made these jobs much less challenging than they would become in the last quarter of the twentieth century. Administrators in the 1950s through the 1980s rarely needed to confront or challenge physicians and largely deferred to their "professional authority." This era was considered a golden age of harmony and mutual success for doctors and hospitals.

The inflation of medical costs that followed the initiation of the federal Medicare program challenged those halcyon days. In 1983, to rein in runaway healthcare costs, Congress passed the Tax Equity and Fiscal Responsibility Act (TEFRA), which instituted a new prospective payment system for hospitals. Diagnosis-related groups (DRGs) fixed reimbursement for a given episode of illness to incent hospitals to control costs, but doctors continued to be paid on a fee-for-service basis. While hospitals searched for ways to reduce patient resource utilization and lengths of stay, doctors practiced as usual, having no economic incentive to support their efforts.

DRGs introduced a significant fault line between doctors and hospitals. For the first time, economic incentives were unaligned, if not in direct conflict, causing an unaccustomed disharmony to spread throughout U.S. hospitals. Institutions hired physicians as utilization advisers, whose job was to pressure colleagues to discharge patients quickly and reduce costs per case. Most doctors were uncomfortable in this role, and the positions were hard to fill. Hospitals ramped up utilization departments and began to second-guess the clinical decisions of their attending doctors. Hallway meetings between administrators and doctors became increasingly tense as the latter complained about the growing infringement on their clinical autonomy. Threats of "economic credentialing" motivated organized medical groups to rail against these new hospital efforts to manage costs.

Events in the last two decades of the twentieth century further alienated doctors and hospitals. Faced with difficult economic realities, many not-for-profit community hospitals were sold to for-profit hospital chains. Comfortable relationships between doctors and local management teams evaporated as corporate management asserted itself in these takeovers. While not all of these transitions were rocky, they heightened physicians' concerns that economics would trump patient care considerations—that management's commitment to shareholder return on investment would interfere with the need to invest in hospital infrastructure. Physicians, perceiving that their places of work were being run for the benefit of shareholders, began to feel less loyal to the hospitals they formerly considered their professional homes. Such feelings became even more prevalent as hospitals began to be bought and sold multiple times to successive investor-owners.

Another major development of the late twentieth century was the emergence of managed care as the economic model du jour. While many physicians were quick to adapt their practices to a capitated payment system, hospitals were not so easy to convert. To ensure they received an adequate number of "covered lives," hospitals began to link themselves to physicians through a variety of mechanisms, including physician–hospital organizations, physician practice management companies, and outright purchase of practices.

These relationships were seldom harmonious. Hospitals had difficulty collaborating with physicians, who usually lacked formal management training and were brought up in the "culture of the expert" that emphasized personal autonomy (Atchison and Bujak 2001). Hospital administrators felt they were "herding cats" in their new relationship with physicians. Doctors observed with derision the failure of most hospitals to run newly purchased physician practices without incurring huge deficits, often in excess of $70,000 per doctor annually. Forced by these losses to divest the practices they had just acquired, many hospitals hesitated to continue physician employment. Some even jettisoned the practices they had purchased at a premium only a few years earlier.

INTO THE TWENTY-FIRST CENTURY

The wreckage left in the wake of the stormy 1990s includes widespread suspicion among physicians regarding hospital administrators' intentions and competence. In tandem, many hospital managers entered the twenty-first century perceiving doctors as their adversaries or as major obstacles to achievement of their organizational goals.

The volatile relationship between doctors and hospitals continues, and a variety of healthcare trends are exacerbating the friction. One trend is the changing locus of physician practice. At the start of the twentieth century, doctors clamored for admission to hospital medical staffs because healthcare institutions were an essential locus of medical work. Hospitals today do not enjoy such status. Many primary care doctors no longer deliver inpatient care. Technological change is also allowing increasing numbers of specialists to practice primarily in their offices or other ambulatory sites. As a result of this decentralization, physicians are becoming less loyal to their community hospitals and less motivated to deliver on the historic citizenship requirements of medical staff membership.

The rapid growth of competition between doctors and hospitals is another trend fraying physician–hospital alignment. As reimbursements decline and overhead costs increase, many physicians are taking over sources of revenue that hospitals have historically claimed. Doctors are investing in outpatient medical facilities and technologies that deliver diagnostic and therapeutic services previously provided by hospitals. Because doctors control patient referrals, they can direct more profitable patients to their own facilities, leaving underinsured or uninsured patients to hospitals. In some parts of the country, doctors are investing in boutique specialty hospitals to divert lucrative revenue streams from local full-service community hospitals. Even when physicians are interested in joining with hospitals to pursue economic goals, they are impeded by huge statutory barriers, including the Stark laws and various anti-kickback statutes at the federal and state levels (see Chapter 12).

Yet another trend aggravating hospital–physician relations is third parties' demands for greater transparency regarding hospital performance. Patients, regulators, politicians, employers, and payers want a safer, higher-quality product from hospitals. These demands are being reinforced by pay-for-performance reimbursement formulas, refusals to pay for "never" events (i.e., preventable quality mishaps), an increasing number of lawsuits claiming hospital negligence, and threats of exclusion from payer networks if performance lags established benchmarks. Hospitals can achieve and publish excellent results only when physicians collaborate with them vigorously. As a result, hospitals are putting ever-increasing demands on their voluntary medical staffs. Physicians, busy and burdened by their own frustrations about the increasingly complex regulatory environment, tend to resent these pressures. As a result, many hospitals are finding that their medical staff members don't have the time or inclination to assist meaningfully in hospital-driven efforts to achieve regulatory compliance or performance targets established unilaterally by payers.

The changing demographics of the physician population add further complexity. Younger physicians are flooding the healthcare workplace, many of whom have different values than their older mentors and eschew the excessive work hours that have long been a hallmark of the medical profession. Greater numbers are looking for part-time options or intend to take leaves of absence for some part of their careers to pursue other interests. The growing number of women practicing medicine may be prompting this trend. Nearly 50 percent of medical school students are female, a notable change from the historic gender ratios in medical education.

If the desire for a more flexible lifestyle is a significant point of friction between physicians and hospitals, so is the consternation of doctors who believe their professional autonomy is under attack. These physicians' angst is palpable as they become increasingly subject to scrutiny and criticism regarding the adequacy of their performance. They feel unreasonably constrained when hospitals push the adoption of clinical pathways, enforce codes of professional conduct, demand that they act as team players, require the use of computerized order entry systems, insist on compliance with national patient safety goals, or urge them to improve performance on core measures promulgated by the government.

The hostility that this "assault" on professional autonomy engenders in some practitioners infects all of their interactions in the hospital. These individuals inflame their colleagues at medical staff meetings in an attempt to get everyone to oppose even the most reasonable efforts by hospitals to gain physician cooperation. Many of these individuals seem to be auditioning for the part of "last angry man" on the medical staff.[3]

Hospitals are not the only targets of this cantankerousness; physicians' sense of alienation is widespread. Some leaders in the field are concerned that the love of practice and commitment that marked previous generations of physicians are eroding, as evidenced by new attitudes toward work; demands for reimbursement for services that used to be uncompensated; and the rise of questionable economic relationships with drug companies, medical device manufacturers, and other industry players. These concerns have prompted the Medical Professionalism Project of the American Board of Internal Medicine (ABIM) Foundation[4] (see Exhibit 1.1).

These factors are only some of the dynamics shaping the healthcare environment as we near the second decade of the twenty-first century. Hospitals are responding with a variety of tactics to shore up their relationships with physicians, many of which are discussed in Chapter 2. Despite the failures of physician employment in the preceding two decades, the most significant response has been the growing employment of physicians by health systems. Physicians, hospitals, and communities believe this arrangement is an answer to many of their needs. We will explore their rationale in Chapter 3. Despite all of the turmoil described above, tight integration of hospitals and doctors is critical if we are to deliver the high-quality, efficient, affordable healthcare this country desperately needs. The proposals unveiled in the following chapters address many of the challenges summarized in Exhibit 1.2 and offer the most promising means of effectively integrating physicians with modern healthcare institutions.

Exhibit 1.1 Medical Professionalism in the New Millennium: A Physician Charter

"Perhaps the principal statement of the ethical code that defines the profession is the Hippocratic Oath—a document authored circa 4th century BC. Given the phenomenal change in medical practice since then, the ABIM Foundation, in collaboration with the ACP Foundation (American College of Physicians) and the European Federation of Internal Medicine (EFIM), published 'Medical Professionalism in the New Millennium: A Physician Charter.'

"The Charter sought not to replace the Hippocratic Oath, but rather to consider the ethical principles that are relevant today, in an environment in which medicine's commitment to the patient is being challenged by external forces of change within our society. The Physician Charter on Medical Professionalism lays out three principles—related to the primacy of patient welfare, to patient autonomy, and to social justice—which are the foundation to the ten commitments that are proposed to guide ethical behavior."

Source: ABIM Foundation (2009).

Exhibit 1.2 A Review of the Forces Straining the Relationship Between Hospitals and Doctors

- The growing migration of physician practice from inpatient to outpatient settings
- Increasing competition between hospitals and private physician practices, especially the development of specialty hospitals, ambulatory

---

surgery centers, outpatient diagnostic centers, and other ambulatory health facilities

- Demands by payers and the public for greater transparency in health-care regarding hospital/physician performance
- Pay-for-performance and bundled-payment reimbursement arrangements
- Encroachment on physician autonomy
- Growth of regulatory requirements for hospitals that can be met only through collaboration with physicians
- Decline of physician interest in the organized medical staff
- Stark laws and other anti-kickback statutes that prevent hospitals from sharing revenues with physicians
- Doctors' increasing interest in manageable lifestyles that are not centered solely on professional work
- Ill will lingering from failed joint ventures, unsuccessful practice acquisitions by hospitals, shared-risk managed care collaborations that were not durable, and short-lived physician–hospital organizations
- Growing use of exclusive contracts by hospitals, which angers some members of the physician community
- Hospitals' efforts to make credentialing and peer review programs more rigorous
- New requirements for hospitals to address disruptive physician behavior

NOTES

1. Discussions of this early work by the American College of Surgeons appear in the following: *Demanding Medical Excellence* by M. Millenson, University of Chicago Press, 1997, pages 143–48; *In Sickness and in Wealth* by R. Stevens, Basic Books, 1989, pages 76–79; and *Health Care Credentialing: A Guide to Innovative Practices* by F. Rozovsky, C. Giles, and M. Kadzielski, Wolters Kluwer, 2007, pages xi–xvii.

2. A description of the current Medicare Conditions of Participation can be found at www.cms.hhs.gov/CFCsAndCOPs.

3. *The Last Angry Man* is a 1959 movie about a cantankerous elderly doctor in Brooklyn. He upholds a lot of values that the present generation in the film seems to have lost.

4. See www.abimfoundation.org/professionalism/charter.shtm.

CHAPTER 2

Toward a Comprehensive Physician Strategy

FOR DECADES, hospital boards have paid little attention to strategies for strengthening relationships with physicians. In times when physicians needed hospitals and were available to hospitals in abundance, these relationships were taken for granted. Physician planning exercises typically revolved around the creation and periodic review of a medical staff development plan—essentially a blueprint for recruiting. As described in Chapter 1, times have changed dramatically. Today, forward-thinking hospitals seeking strong connections with their physician communities must create comprehensive strategies to build them.

A PHYSICIAN DEVELOPMENT PLAN VERSUS A COMPREHENSIVE STRATEGY

Most hospitals are familiar with the process of assessing their community's current and future needs for health professionals. The concept of a medical staff development plan evolved decades ago to create a context for discussions with the physician community about service and access. Physician development plans also allow hospitals to legally close certain departments or specialties to new applicants without running afoul of antitrust and related laws. Hospitals conduct formal community needs assessments to inform physician recruiting strategies, justify stipends and signing bonuses, and convince reluctant medical staff members of the need to recruit.

The physician shortage—already problematic in many areas of the country and looming in every community—has injected new urgency into the process of planning for recruitment. Our experience, however, has convinced us that quantifying recruitment needs is only a preliminary step in the process of crafting a comprehensive physician strategy. Additional steps must be taken to retain staff, make the medical community attractive to potential new applicants, ensure excellent communication among members of the healthcare community, and keep physicians engaged in hospital concerns.

Most critical to the development of a comprehensive strategy is creation of a plan that not only meets the community's physician staffing needs but also aligns physicians with the hospital to the extent needed to fulfill the hospital's mission and the community's desire for care coordinated across service sites. The process of generating a comprehensive strategy creates a context in which hospitals can see employment as important to engagement.

THE DIFFERENCE BETWEEN A MEDICAL STAFF AND A PHYSICIAN PRACTICE COMMUNITY

Medical care has been migrating away from hospitals for over a decade. First we saw diagnostic procedures move to the ambulatory arena, and then simple surgeries and endoscopic procedures moved off-site. This trend is continuing. Increasingly, primary care physicians are using hospitalists to tend to their patients after admission. Because many insurance companies require all physicians to maintain hospital privileges, most general internists and family practitioners still belong to their local hospital's medical staff. We believe, however, that this requirement will give way to pressure from primary care providers, many who see little value in maintaining a hospital affiliation. Once insurance companies relax their policies, we expect large-scale withdrawal of primary care physicians from hospital staffs.

Primary care doctors are not the only group attenuating their connections to hospitals. Specialists are also moving their practices to the outpatient arena. The use of private ambulatory surgery centers, endoscopy suites, urgent care offices, and increasingly sophisticated in-office diagnostic testing facilities has prompted this shift. Driven by new technology and the finances of private practice, specialists, like primary care doctors, are spending less time at the community hospital. The work of the traditional, organized medical staff is becoming less relevant to them, making apathy one of the greatest challenges medical staff leaders face today.

For these reasons, we prefer to understand the physician-related strategic efforts of hospitals not within the narrow frame of reference of "our relationship with the organized medical staff" but within the broader frame of reference of "our relationship with our practice community." In addition to formal members of the staff, this broader concept includes all physicians in the hospital service area whose referral patterns affect community health and system success, including those aligned with competitors. The jargon of the *practice community* helps us appreciate the community's complexity, whereas *medical staff* jargon invites us to erroneously perceive the staff as unitary and homogeneous in needs and perspectives. The typical elected or appointed leadership of organized medical staffs cannot represent the full range of physician interests that hospital management and the board must address.

THE HEART OF ANY COMPREHENSIVE STRATEGY—A DETAILED PRACTICE-BY-PRACTICE ANALYSIS

The traditional medical staff development plan provided a limited set of data concerning physicians. It typically assessed the age and

Exhibit 2.1 Practice Identification and Contact Tracking

Specialty	Practice Name	Geography Covered	Number of Practitioners	Growth/ Replacement Plans Within the Practice	Last Contact, Promises, Next Contact

retirement plans of staff practitioners and matched this information with data concerning community growth rates and service needs. This information was reviewed in concert with the hospital's strategic plan to determine recruitment targets needed to meet to maintain or extend market share.

These data continue to be important and provide an opportunity to learn about a hospital's practice community, but an effective development plan needs to consider more than age and retirement plans. For instance, which local physician practices have internal strategic plans? Are they synergistic with the hospital's goals? Do physicians in the community have expectations of the hospital that it may not be aware of? Are there opportunities to work together to meet mutual needs? (*What could the hospital and you do together to strengthen your practice?* is an excellent question to pose in a medical staff survey.) Is the hospital's communication approach working well with each practice, or does it need to be improved? The answers to these and many other relevant questions can be determined if the periodic medical staff development survey process is elevated to produce a comprehensive survey of physician practices and needs.

Exhibit 2.2 Practice-by-Practice Strategic Analysis

	Current	Anticipated in Two Years	Anticipated in Five Years
Practice history (date of founding, critical milestones in practice evolution)		—	—
Practice leader(s)			
Economic model (i.e., how is income generated—fee for service only, managed care, ancillary ownership?)			
Primary hospital administrative contact			
Current economic integration/ competition with hospital; economic opportunities to increase alignment			
Personal/emotional connection with hospital; opportunities			
Practice concerns			
Practice needs			
Preferred communication approach			
Hospital's alignment strategy			

Exhibits 2.1 and 2.2 can be used to organize a great deal of data and create a scaffold for complex and sophisticated planning. If your institution currently has a contact database or relationship management database, you may be able to customize your existing software to create data fields that mirror these headings.

THE EPHEMERAL GOAL OF HOSPITAL–PHYSICIAN ALIGNMENT

Given the changes in medical practice outlined in Chapter 1, hospitals need to engage their local physicians much more than most local physicians need to engage hospitals. The imbalance in this equation fills hospital executives with understandable consternation and keeps them reflecting on how they align with "their" doctors. Assuming alignment is the "natural state," or demanding alignment as though it is physicians' moral obligation, will not work. To achieve alignment, a hospital must leverage its understanding of physician needs to create a viable value proposition with each provider or provider group.

There are 11 strategies critical to the process of creating alignment. The first five are essential regardless of the economic model on which alignment is based; the next six pertain to economic models that are different than the traditional arrangement between hospitals and doctors (i.e., complete independence). Physician employment emerges as a critical option, supporting our thesis.

Essential Strategies

Service

Countless surveys have affirmed that physicians most desire *service*, defined as *ease of practice*, from the hospitals in which they work. Is the hospital user-friendly for physicians? Is it efficient? Can doctors obtain what they need to care for their patients without undue effort? Is physician parking convenient? Is equipment readily available? Are reports easily retrievable? Are the nurses competent? Are there sufficient operating room slots? *Service* also extends to patient satisfaction. What do patients say to their physicians? Do they complain about the hospital or thank their doctors for choosing to work there? Without adequate service, hospitals will find creating an effective strategy for alignment virtually impossible.

Numerous tactical initiatives can improve the quality of service provided to physicians. For example, putting performance expectations in exclusive contracts (e.g., specific report turnaround times from hospital-based radiologists) can ensure appropriate service. Some hospitals have created operating councils to bring key physicians and administrators together in specific service lines (more on this in Chapter 13). One purpose of these councils is to address ways of making the service line more user-friendly for physicians who underpin its success.

Whatever the technique, keep in mind that soliciting input from physicians but failing to act on this information is counterproductive. Such failures only reinforce physicians' perception that hospitals are poor partners and administrators are untrustworthy.

Communication

Despite the abundance of literature emphasizing communication as a critical element in any successful organization, physicians still routinely complain about inadequate communication with hospitals. The historic approach to communication with physicians has been through meetings, which is becoming less viable as demands on physicians' time increases. Consider using technology for communication, such as dedicated and secure websites, e-mail, faxes, recorded messages, newsletters, personal letters, phones, and even podcasts. Ask key physicians about their preferred form of communication; they are more likely to pay attention to messages delivered in a manner they have chosen.

In the world of hospitals and physicians, successful communication involves attention to five issues:

1. *Inclusiveness*: Physicians are sensitive to being informed of organizational decisions after the fact. They are rightly suspect of requests for input when decisions appear to have already been made and the request seems no more than a wish for them to acquiesce. Postponing decision making to include physicians may seem cumbersome to hospital administrators,

but it is usually worth the extra time. Although most physicians lack administrative sophistication, they often provide valuable feedback. In addition, most doctors will more readily accept a decision they disagree with if they have had a chance to provide input. The message for hospital managers is to *include*, not merely *inform*. For example, administrators send a different message if they include physician leaders early in the hospital's periodic strategic planning process instead of asking them for comments on a strategic planning document that has already been drafted.

2. *Outreach*: If we consider on-call coverage, phone calls, and documentation, physicians generally work 10- to 14-hour days. They have little time, and even less patience, for the meetings central to administrative life. To involve physicians, develop a liaison staff that can reach out to explain administrative issues, harvest ideas and concerns, and follow up. Some hospitals have employed a physician ombudsperson to perform this function, while others use staff from their medical affairs offices. Some assign a person from the executive management team to carry out this activity with each practice important to the hospital's success. Yet others have created a physician cabinet or council of key community physicians who meet regularly with the hospital CEO to ensure that effective dialogue and outreach are occurring.

3. *Personal commitment*: Physicians respond more to personal commitments from senior executives than they do to vague, bureaucratic pronouncements. "We're circulating our new strategic plan" is a much less satisfying communication to a physician than "I am personally committed to achieving 'X' within the next 12 months."

4. *Responsiveness*: From a physician's perspective, the test of any communication strategy is not words but results. Management's credibility rests on its ability to demonstrate that it can put words into action. Even when immediate action is impossible,

as is often the case, hospital leaders need to articulate a project plan that promises specific actions by specific times.

5. *Scope*: Communication need not be an "even-handed" process. Hospital managers should devote energy and effort toward effective communication with key practices because it is more important than communicating with practices that have little impact on the hospital's success. Quarterly visits to targeted physician practices by a member of the senior management team may be useful, but this person may not be able to visit every member of the medical staff. Hospital management may also find value in thinking beyond physicians and considering communication strategies with office managers or practice executive directors.

Physician Leadership

Physicians seem to have a fundamental distrust of executives who have not undergone the training, professional induction, and licensing required to practice medicine. In the best of circumstances, their distrust fades away; we've found, however, that it rarely does. Who, then, can lead physicians? If they are amenable to being led at all, leadership must be assigned to another physician. Perhaps this dynamic will disappear in generations to come, but for now it is something hospital executives need to live with and address effectively.

The implication of this cultural chasm between physicians and hospital executives is that hospitals must develop physician leaders capable of bridging the divide. Initially, in the late 1980s and early 1990s, physicians close to retirement would take on this function, assuming a usually ill-defined role as vice president for medical affairs (VPMA). In the absence of clearly defined duties, these physicians would do their best to serve as ambassadors, shuttling between the hospital executive suite and the physicians' dining room. While this ambassadorship helped maintain harmonious relations, physicians and executives rarely collaborated to design creative solutions to challenges in care delivery.

As the complexity of hospital operations increases, the VPMA job is becoming more complicated, as are the credentialing and peer review duties formally assigned to the medical staff. Successful hospitals are expanding the role of the VPMA and devoting substantial resources to training additional physician leaders on the organized medical staff. Today's physician leaders must understand the complexities of healthcare delivery in considerable depth and be able to move beyond ambassadorship to negotiate durable solutions to complex problems. Local physicians can be trained for this role or recruited from an ever-growing national pool of trained physician executives.

In addition to formal leaders, cultivation of informal leaders—local physicians who appreciate the complexity of the healthcare enterprise and have demonstrated a willingness to collaborate with the hospital—is essential. Their practices become the nucleus of a community of aligned physicians.

Physician Engagement Around Higher Values

Demand for productivity and adequate reimbursement, coupled with frustrations about the logistics of today's practice environment, threaten the heart of physician culture. In the past, professionalism, commitment to the community, and a focus on the patient ensured high public regard for physicians. Sadly, evidence suggests that this regard is not what it once was. However, we are convinced that old-fashioned values of commitment and service are alive or at least latent, obscured by the pressures and frustrations previously mentioned. In this context, hospital leaders—physicians and nonphysicians alike—face the challenge of engaging everyone involved in the healthcare enterprise in a dialogue about values. Such dialogue promotes mutual commitments to higher aspirations and the alignment of short- and long-term goals and plans with those commitments.

Joe Bujak (2008) has written eloquently about the need for physicians and hospital leaders to move beyond talking about details and dollars and engage in probing conversations about deeper questions: Why are we in this profession? What matters most to our communities? What is the measure of a professional life well lived? Dr. Bujak has found that such conversations can lead to a sense of interdependence and commitment that facilitates the solution of more technical problems. We elaborate on this point in Chapter 9 in our discussion of group practice culture.

We have led many retreats that bring together community board members, physicians, and administrators to discuss these higher goals and raise the level of dialogue above parochial concerns. Our experience echoes that of Dr. Bujak. The goal of hospital–physician alignment is more readily achieved when such discussions create a realistic vision of a preferred future for all parties—one grounded in fundamental values of service and professionalism.

Recruitment and Retention

In his book *Good to Great*, Jim Collins (2001, 13) asserts that a company's success depends on "getting the right people on the bus." This concept is every bit as critical to a hospital's physician strategy. Effective recruitment results from more than a simple credentials check. Many questions must be kept in mind, including the following:

- Is this physician likely to stay in the community? (This question may bring up issues about family or cultural fit.)
- Will this physician invest in the success of the healthcare enterprise in this community (versus simply the success of his or her own practice)?
- Does he or she appreciate the importance of the hospital to the community?
- Does this doctor have communication and problem-solving skills that would be an asset to the organization?
- Does this physician have leadership interests or skills?

A rigorous recruitment strategy will increase the chances of finding physicians amenable to alignment, but it does little to answer the two critical questions hospitals face regarding retention: How do they distinguish physicians who are willing and able to work with them, and what do they do about physicians associated with the hospital who seem to have no interest in collaboration?

An *intended practice plan* can be used to determine the answers to these questions. This document can be completed by medical staff applicants along with the traditional application forms. The information it requests is used to assess whether a practitioner is likely to be an asset to the institution. The following are examples of questions included in an intended practice plan:

- Do you intend to admit or refer patients for admission to this hospital?
- Do you intend to refer patients to this hospital for diagnostic testing?
- Do you intend to consult with the specialists on this medical staff?
- Are you planning to participate in the hospital's emergency department on-call schedule?
- Are you willing to serve on medical staff committees and take on other medical staff citizenship roles?
- If your answer to any of these questions is "no," how do you intend to help this hospital promote its mission in the community?

The intended practice plan provides a window into the intentions of a potential medical staff member. It sets the stage for important conversations about interdependence and mutual commitment. The physician's future behavior can be compared to his or her responses to the plan questions, and this comparison can form a basis for discussion on whether long-term medical staff membership is warranted.

Options for Economic Alignment

Infrastructure Support
While the Stark laws are strict in terms of what hospitals can offer to independent members of their medical staff, these regulations

have recently been relaxed to allow hospital support through the computerization of health records. Despite this change of policy, evidence suggests that most hospitals have not taken advantage of the opportunity to work closely with physicians to promote computerized information sharing. Hospitals also have opportunities to provide services that many privately practicing physicians need, such as purchasing, human resources support, billing services, telecommunications services, and biohazardous waste management. While Stark regulations require that market prices be charged for many of these services, a win/win equation can still be created by customizing service packages to the unique environment of the physician's office. In some cases, charges for these services can be moderated by taking advantage of the economies of scale gained through group purchasing.

Co-branding and Marketing

"A brand is a promise," the saying goes. When a hospital or health system has succeeded in creating a strong local brand and is trusted by its community, it can invite local physicians to join forces and share that brand. Physicians can then benefit from marketing/public relations efforts that support their practices via association with the hospital's reputation and resources.

Employment

As we will describe in depth in the following two chapters, both independent, hospital-based physicians and doctors practicing ambulatory medicine are seeking employment with hospitals as never before. Paradoxically, the same physicians who cling to autonomy and want to escape hospital work nonetheless seek organizational shelter as employees. Hospital employment offers physicians stability, significant relief from the administrative burdens of practice, and an opportunity to be a part of a system with a longitudinal commitment to the community. Employment nullifies most of the constraints of the Stark laws, enabling hospital support of physician practices limited only by the hospital's need to create a sustainable business model for physician employment. To achieve long-term success in such an environment, however, physicians have to sacrifice significant autonomy and commit to organizational citizenship, neither of which is easy to do.

Exclusive Contracting

Single-specialty groups, particularly hospital-based groups, are often engaged in collaborative work via exclusive contracts. Local physicians may see such contracts as anticompetitive, but they are legally permissible on the basis of the argument that they ensure access, continuity, and quality of care to a hospital's patient community. In our experience, exclusive contracts usually do little more than describe clinical and coverage duties, clarify reimbursement, and then go into legal boilerplate. In these cases, the opportunity for building deeper structural alignment and more rigorous expectations for quality and safety is squandered. We recommend embedding specific leadership duties in the scope of contractual services—duties within the group, and duties supporting the hospital's service and quality initiatives. These contracts should also include tailored performance expectations and specify metrics that will be taken to ensure compliance.

Traditionally restricted to hospital-based practitioners such as radiologists, anesthesiologists, pathologists, and emergency room doctors, exclusive contracts today are aligning a much broader array of specialties with hospitals. Examples include hospitalists, cardiothoracic surgeons, neurosurgeons, pain management specialists, and trauma surgeons. When legally justified, such arrangements are an excellent means of ensuring that the involved practitioners and the hospital establish mutual commitments and codify them in contractual language.

Joint Ventures

Joint ventures between physicians and hospitals have acquired a bad reputation over the years. A good business opportunity is not necessarily a good joint venture opportunity, and joint ventures alone are not an alignment strategy. However, this vehicle can be used to synergize physicians and hospitals economically. Hospitals should consider pursuing a joint venture in the following situations:

- When they are working with mature physician groups capable of understanding the work involved in long-term strategic partnerships
- When collaboration would tightly bond providers at risk of moving into a competitive posture
- When the investment in strategic partnership offers both parties opportunities for business growth that would offset the revenue loss that results from "sharing the pie"

Like exclusive contracts, successful joint ventures should not split revenue on the basis of simple economic formulas. They can be carefully structured to engage physicians in the creation of innovative strategies and the pursuit of better quality and efficiency and to commit them to long-term community service.

Gainsharing

Gainsharing, which financially rewards physicians for successful participation in various hospital-driven efforts, had been deemed illegal by the federal government for well over a decade. In recent years, Washington policymakers have been reconsidering this position and now permit limited gainsharing activity.

One use of the term refers to efforts at engaging physicians in cost containment (such as reducing the cost of implantable devices). If physicians participate in these efforts, hospitals reward them by reinvesting savings into areas that help their practice (e.g., by adding operating rooms). In this example, physicians are not rewarded financially in a direct sense but are rewarded with expedited ease of practice.

A bolder example of gainsharing involves trial projects by the Centers for Medicare & Medicaid Services that financially reward physicians who drive improved performance by participating in initiatives that simultaneously increase quality and reduce cost. These programs are under high regulatory scrutiny and should not be undertaken without the assistance of experienced legal counsel.

Another recent example of this type of gainsharing is the permission the Office of Inspector General (OIG) gave one health system to share pay-for-performance dollars with the physicians who helped generate them. In this case, the health system had a contract with a third-party payer that provided financial rewards for reaching specified performance targets. The hospital engaged members of its medical staff to achieve the targeted goals, and the hospital received bonus money under its contract with the payer when it met those targets. The OIG created narrow criteria that, if met, would allow this money to be shared with physicians without raising a red flag to regulators.

CONCLUSION

Not all physicians in a practice community will be interested in close alignment with their local hospital. Further, all physicians are not of equal strategic value to a community hospital (e.g., a general surgeon versus a dermatologist), nor should a hospital necessarily engage all available providers, as some may fail to meet fundamental standards of quality, service, or civility.

In view of these realities, hospitals need to adopt a careful strategy that targets physician engagement and is marked by egalitarianism and an openness to work with all who are interested in a collaborative relationship; are able to address unmet community/hospital needs; and meet organizational standards for quality work, citizenship, and service. Once this strategy is in place, hospitals need a comprehensive plan for pursuing strengthened relations with physicians (see Exhibit 2.3). Greater alignment of interests, service contracts, and employment are essential to this effort.

These suggested modes of engagement do not guarantee results, but they do point hospitals in the right direction. In hospitals'

Exhibit 2.3 A Comprehensive List of Tactics for Promoting Hospital–Physician Alignment

Hospitals use the following approaches to strengthen alliances with private practice physicians or otherwise create legal and economic relationships with willing physicians.

Strengthen Hospital Alliances with Physicians in Private Practice

- Assist private practices in their recruitment efforts
- Provide practice support where legally possible (e.g., implementation of electronic health records)
- Support common marketing and branding initiatives
- Engage these physicians through structured dialogue and appreciative inquiry[1]
- Engage key physicians in the redesign of hospital operations to minimize burdens on physician time
- Provide support for physician practice strategic planning
- Promote excellent communication:
    - Maintain an ombudsperson to handle physician concerns
    - Create a physician advisory council or cabinet
    - Create a medical staff website
    - Other tactics include practice visits by administrators, creation of a council of office managers, invitations to private office staff to tour hospital facilities, and excellent orientations to hospital services for doctors and staffs
- Create a professional medical staff that is more inclusive than the organized medical staff and includes all community physicians seeking identification with the hospital
- Support and underwrite local continuing medical education
- Publicly celebrate accomplishments of physicians on staff or in the community
- Develop a system to thank physicians for exceptional service

Establish Relationships by Contract

- Employ physician managers, such as medical directors

(Continued on following page)

- Contract for specific clinical services (e.g., study interpretation, emergency department coverage, committee work)
- Expand exclusive contracts
- Employ physicians directly
- Use an intended practice plan (this type of plan is a "quasi" contract— typically not legally binding)

Strengthen the Organized Medical Staff
- Create a leadership university or equivalent
- Engage in active succession planning
- Employ tactics to increase social capital (e.g., golf outings, dinner dances)
- Use all technologies to communicate effectively with the medical staff (i.e., do not rely on poorly attended meetings)
- Make peer review collegial and eliminate the culture of shame and blame
- Help physicians use individual performance reports to secure pay-for-performance benefits from insurers
- Give lots of service awards to recognize the efforts of medical staff
- Avoid divisiveness over medical staff categories by redesigning where necessary

struggle to create more symbiotic connections with the physician community, contractual relationships are most successful because they spell out mutual commitments with clarity and firm obligation. Of the contractual relationships (employment, exclusive contracts, joint ventures), employment maximizes alignment, which is one explanation for the renewed welcome hospitals have for physicians as employees.

In the next two chapters, we will expand on the forces driving renewed employment and factors essential to successful physician employment. We will then proceed by describing the conceptual and operational leap from simple employment to group practice formation that hospitals must take to create value on an ongoing basis.

NOTE

1. These communication approaches are described in *Better Communication for Better Care: Mastering Physician-Administrator Collaboration* by Kenneth H. Cohn, MD, FACS, Health Administration Press, 2005.

CHAPTER 3

The Second Wave of Physician Employment

AS DISCUSSED IN CHAPTER 2, hospital employment of physicians as an alignment strategy is increasing. Numerous factors are driving this trend, including the hostile business climate surrounding the private practice of medicine and the changing value propositions of younger physicians. In combination, these factors are inexorably shifting doctors away from the traditional private practice of medicine. The majority of physicians in the United States today are in professional employment relationships of some type. This dramatic upswing in employment is setting the stage for hospital-led group formation.

FACTORS DRIVING PHYSICIANS TO SEEK HOSPITAL EMPLOYMENT

The Dim Business Prospects of Private Practice

Year after year, doctors' offices face new regulatory burdens, the costs of new technology, rising malpractice premiums, the expense of accommodating the byzantine rules of multiple payers, and salary increases for employees who are becoming ever more scarce and difficult to recruit. Once able to attend to practice management and clinical practice simultaneously, more and more physicians are having to hire skilled (and expensive) office personnel to supervise these mounting complexities.

Even as office expenses grow, payers are becoming increasingly effective at resisting physician demand for increased reimbursement. The consolidation of healthcare payers across the nation has given them enormous market power in this respect. The country's largest payer, the federal government, regularly issues threats of draconian cuts to the Medicare physician payment schedule. Most doctors feel they are working harder to earn less. Government antitrust laws prevent doctors from working in concert to improve payment schedules. Unable to raise their rates unilaterally, doctors are having difficulty maintaining adequate office staff and facilities, investing in expensive healthcare technology, offering salary guarantees to prospective partners, and satisfying their own income expectations.

The technology issue is particularly daunting. Doctors are under increasing external pressure to computerize patient records. The quality and safety arguments in favor of electronic health records are compelling, but the costs of conversion—including hardware, software, training, and inevitable upgrades—are higher than most solo and small group offices can afford.

Under these constraints, more and more small office practices are becoming nonviable. The physicians who own these practices are demanding hospital employment, threatening to leave their communities and seek opportunities elsewhere if refused. A clear indication of the sorry financial prospects of most physician practices is that today (as opposed to common practice only a decade ago) almost no one is offering to pay "goodwill" for the acquisition of a physician practice. (We will touch on the concept of goodwill later.)

The Toll of Private Practice on Professional Life

Most private physician practices are small business operations. In the past, physicians both managed office business and provided patient care. In recent years, the entrepreneurial drive of many doctors has been extinguished by the reality of ever-increasing operational complexity. Eager to hang up the mantle of business operator and focus exclusively on clinical care, an increasing number of doctors are asking hospitals to buy or assume their practices. Most of these physicians are in the last third of their career and have robust practices but wish to decelerate their professional life as they near retirement. The cohort of physicians approaching retirement age is substantial; in 2006, approximately one-third of the country's physicians were aged 55 or older (Croasdale 2006; U.S. Department of Health and Human Services 2006).

Value Shifts Among Younger Physicians

As younger physicians come to dominate the clinical workforce, so will their generation's values and priorities. Preferences of recent residency graduates and those in the medical education pipeline include

- greater balance between the commitments to work and home life,
- increased opportunity to pursue personal interests outside of medicine,
- employment opportunities that do not involve running a private entrepreneurial business,
- group practice arrangements with "reasonable" call schedules and part-time practice options,
- stable income based on national benchmarks (rather than the salary uncertainty of private practice), and
- clinical settings that use established electronic medical records.[1]

These preferences translate into increased interest in employment opportunities. In a survey of students at Duke University

Medical School, 74 percent of respondents indicated a desire to practice in an employment relationship rather than in traditional private practice (E. Lister and M. Maloney, unpublished data).

Hospitals are not the sole providers of employment opportunities; many private physician practices start new physicians as employees. They usually expect, however, that these new colleagues will transition to a private practice model. In contrast, hospitals can offer long-term employment. In addition, hospitals are more likely to offer reasonable call schedules, a larger number of colleagues, electronic medical records similar to those used by new doctors during their training, part-time practice or leave of absence options, and financial stability—all linked to nationally competitive salary offers.

DRIVERS OF REEMERGING HOSPITAL INTEREST IN PHYSICIAN EMPLOYMENT

The Eroding Physician–Hospital Compact

Traditional and mutually acceptable obligations between hospitals and doctors (what Chris Argryis [1960] called the "psychological contract," and Jack Silversin and Mary Jane Kornacki [2000] later referred to as the "physician compact") are dissolving rapidly. As doctors struggle under the burdens of private practice, they are resisting, with increasing frequency and tenacity, routine responsibilities such as committee assignments, assumption of medical staff leadership roles, and attendance at staff meetings. Further, many hospitals are finding they can no longer expect the members of their medical staff to voluntarily provide services once considered citizenship obligations. Doctors are now asking for payment to provide these services.

Many doctors are also unwilling to continue providing unpaid emergency room coverage. Where they have the market power to do so, some practitioners are demanding compensation for call services that hospital administrators find unfair and unsustainable.

Equally beleaguered hospital leadership teams may come to regard these physicians as extortionists. Even hospitals willing to pay are struggling to find doctors amenable to providing essential call or coverage services. Many physicians simply don't want to suffer the lifestyle impact or malpractice exposure that results from being openly available to the hospital emergency department. Once hospitals concede that they need to provide physicians with some form of payment to motivate them to fulfill needed clinical services, they will inevitably consider more seriously the advantages of a fully employed physician workforce.

What is the connection between employment and fulfillment of these tasks? An employed doctor can be assigned a schedule of tasks that encompasses emergency care appropriately and comprehensively and is codified by contract. If they are managed appropriately, such doctors are likely to work more productively toward hospital goals than would private physicians offered monetary enticements piecemeal for only one slice of clinical activity.

Inadequate Supply of Physicians

Hospitals are having more and more difficulty meeting their physician workforce needs. In part, this shortage can be attributed to a greater number of doctors focusing their work hours in the outpatient setting. This trend started over a decade ago in the primary care specialties, when physicians began to shift procedures from inpatient to outpatient settings. Through the 1980s and 1990s, managed care operations challenged the need for hospitalization for one condition after another. The medical community realized that many procedures previously performed by habit in the hospital could, with greater efficiency and diminished expense, be performed in the outpatient environment. Physicians began taking ownership of these ambulatory operations, which ranged from small-scale office-based lab and X-ray facilities to large-scale ambulatory surgery and freestanding diagnostic centers, allowing them to supplement the income they generated from professional fees with income generated from technical fees.

Other economic issues also underpin this trend. Primary care doctors make more money when they spend their time in the office than when they travel to see patients in the hospital. Similarly, many specialists are more compelled to spend time on more lucrative outpatient procedures (e.g., cosmetic surgery or colonoscopy) than on complex inpatient cases. Some specialists are choosing to limit their inpatient privileges to avoid treating cases that may demand a lot of time and effort. For example, a plastic surgeon may not want privileges to operate on decubitus ulcers or to treat hand injuries; a gastroenterologist may drop privileges to treat bleeding varices; and an obstetrician-gynecologist may decide to opt out of practicing obstetrics. To compensate for these defections from inpatient care, hospitals have resorted to employing their own workforce of medical and surgical hospitalists, laborists, and proceduralists.

An even greater challenge facing hospitals is the growing national shortage of physicians.[2] The shortage has been and will be particularly acute in primary care disciplines as a result of economic trends that reward specialists for performing procedures more than they reward family practitioners and internists for prevention or longitudinal treatment of chronic diseases. These economic considerations have helped drive career choices among medical students away from primary care and into specialties. Other factors prompting predictions of a physician shortage in the decades ahead include

- national population growth;
- the tide of aging baby boomers, who will be high consumers of medical services and require an increasing volume of physician visits per capita;
- decreased physician productivity resulting from the lifestyle preferences of younger physicians;
- decreased physician productivity likely to result from the increasing number of women doctors in the workforce

(women physicians historically have worked fewer hours than their male counterparts and are more likely to take a leave of absence sometime during their working career); and

- the imminent retirement of physicians of the baby-boom generation.

In the early 1990s, the consensus was that the country was producing too many doctors. During this time, the Council on Graduate Medical Education (COGME) was advocating for fewer residency training slots, and Congress capped the number of residency positions funded by Medicare. However, by the turn of the millennium, pundits were publishing revised figures warning of a looming physician shortage. While the projections vary widely, some studies predict that the nation may be short nearly 200,000 doctors by 2020. In a significant about-face, several years ago COGME urged Congress to remove the Medicare graduate medical education funding cap and exhorted the nation's medical schools to increase annual class size by 15 percent. The Association of American Medical Colleges went a step further and called for 30 percent more U.S. medical school graduates annually. Despite this call to action, the nation lacks the faculty, training resources, and, in particular, the graduate medical education positions to accommodate such an increase any time soon.

Not everyone agrees that we need more doctors. Most of those who challenge the idea of a shortage suggest that redistribution of America's physicians would remedy the problem. This argument is not without merit, but it belies the fact that we have no mechanism for enacting such redistribution.

To ensure their ability to provide necessary services in their communities, many hospitals are aggressively hiring physicians in low-supply, high-demand specialties. While most small private physician groups cannot afford to bring on additional members until patient demand breaks even with costs, hospitals can subsidize employed physicians on their payrolls as patient demand grows, giving them a competitive advantage.

Recruitment will only become harder in the years ahead if the physician shortage worsens as predicted. Hospitals unable to accommodate graduates or local physicians seeking employment will see increasing defection from their physician community. By employing physicians now, hospitals can round out their staffs before shortages become acute.

Competition Between Hospitals and Physicians

Competition between hospitals and private practitioners is growing, largely as a result of the increase in physician ownership of ambulatory resources mentioned earlier. Hospitals, which historically "owned" the ancillary and technical revenue streams, are experiencing this competition as betrayal. They also make the legitimate argument that these lost revenues are essential to underwriting money-losing services of critical importance to the community (e.g., emergency care, obstetrics, burn care, care for the uninsured). Physician-owners of ancillary revenue streams, however, believe that competition with hospitals is fair under the rules of a market economy and that, merely by virtue of their size, hospitals must have some other way of meeting community needs.

Significant competition can create great friction within the hospital medical staff and sour working relationships, both among physicians and between doctors and management. When these relationships become rocky, engaging doctors in the advancement of the hospital's goals becomes difficult. When physicians are employed, on the other hand, their financial interests are automatically aligned with those of the hospital.

The Imperative of Better Clinical and Operational Performance

Payers and regulators are imposing ever-increasing demands on hospitals for quality, safety, transparency, and service. Pay for performance, now a common practice, links hospital reimbursement to those demands. Three other payer initiatives are also reinforcing that link. The first is a refusal to pay for *never events*—care delivery errors that are considered preventable. The second is what the Centers for Medicare & Medicaid Services calls *value-based pricing*—a strategy that prices products on the basis of their demand. The third is an approach called *bundled payment*—one payment for an episode of patient care (includes preadmission, inpatient, and post-discharge care).

Clinicians in private practice are often unmotivated to actively help their hospital meet pay-for-performance goals or collaborate on the treatment protocols required to receive bundled payments. Likewise, traditional medical staff executive committees are not formally mandated to be involved in payment matters and are unlikely to support pay-for-performance goals that are often a source of contention among medical staff members.

Employed physicians, in contrast, can be contractually bound to meet performance expectations set by the hospital. Employed physicians can be given economic incentives to achieve ambitious quality targets, improve patient satisfaction, and enhance the reputation of the institution. In the highly competitive healthcare world, these important advantages accrue to hospitals with significant numbers of employed physicians. We elaborate on these issues in chapters 10 and 11.

HOSPITAL PRACTICE ACQUISITION VERSUS DIRECT EMPLOYMENT

As described earlier, the 1980s and 1990s saw hospitals in many parts of the country engage in a feeding frenzy over the acquisition of physician practices. At that time, premiums were paid to physicians for goodwill, making practice purchase exceedingly expensive.[3] When practices were acquired, however, physician performance expectations were not articulated, and the productivity anticipated by the hospital was not achieved. Losses mounted, and the physician employment strategy was deemed a failure.

This experience has made many hospital CEOs and boards averse to practice acquisition. However, when a community physician who is valuable to the hospital requests employment for the reasons articulated at the beginning of this chapter, the hospital usually has little choice other than to acquire the practice or see that physician exit the hospital community. Chapter 4 explains how practices can be acquired without experiencing the difficulties of previous decades.

Reluctant to incur the risks and complexities of being a physician employer, many hospitals offer only temporary or transitional employment to new physicians. Employment is offered as a recruitment incentive, with the idea that once practices are stable and self-supporting, physicians will spin off into traditional private practice. From our perspective, this strategy embraces all of the costs of start-up and sacrifices all of the long-term gains we describe in this book. Short-term employment of this sort is an expensive recruitment strategy and does not answer the ongoing need for the close alignment of physician and hospital interests that can improve efficiency, quality, and service.

If hiring physicians is becoming an essential alignment strategy, how can hospitals travel this path successfully? Chapter 4 addresses the first step to creating a successful employed group practice—mastering the basics of employment.

NOTES

1. Numerous recruiting firms regularly survey the preferences of physicians in training. For example, see the 2008 Survey of Final Year Medical Residents conducted by Merritt Hawkins & Associates at www.merritthawkins.com/pdf/2008-mha-survey-medical-residents.pdf.

2. A survey performed by The Physician's Foundation and Merritt Hawkins & Associates in October 2008 found that 49 percent of physicians—more than 150,000 doctors nationwide—said that over the next three years they plan to

reduce the number of patients they see or stop practicing entirely. In that same time frame:

- 11 percent—more than 35,000 doctors nationwide—said they plan to retire,
- 13 percent said they plan to seek a job in a nonclinical healthcare setting, which would remove them from active patient care,
- 20 percent said they will cut back on the number of patients they see, and
- 10 percent said they will work part time.

3. *Goodwill* is a nebulous construct having to do with a physician's reputation in the community and the assumption that this social standing translates into a tangible business asset. It was usually estimated by taking some multiple (.5 to 1.5) of net practice income.

CHAPTER 4

Physician Employment: Getting the Basics Right

ALTHOUGH FULLY INTEGRATED GROUP PRACTICES are more structurally complex and therefore more difficult to manage, they enjoy significant advantages over portfolios of disaggregated employed physicians. Acquiring the skills needed to employ an effective physician workforce is the first step to successfully managing that complexity. Group practice success stems from the development of those skills, as detailed in the following chapters. What is this set of basic skills?

VENUES FOR EVERY PHYSICIAN PREFERENCE

To be successful, health systems must attract physicians who are "aligned enough" to support the enterprise with referrals for admission, lab and diagnostic testing, or surgery. We see physician employment not as a goal in itself but as a critical element of the formula for success. "Enough physicians who are good enough and aligned enough" is one way of expressing this formula.

If employment—or group practice formation—is a means to achieving health system success rather than an end in itself, a hospital's physician strategy should not involve driving or forcing physicians into employment. Rather, the challenge is to create an optimal practice venue for all physicians interested in collaboration, with hospital employment as an attractive option. Some still may want an old-fashioned, small practice; others may want to explore the possibility of concierge medicine; and yet others may want to be part of an unaffiliated group. Hospitals should be adept at accommodating multiple models of engagement.

To prevent tension from building between employed physicians and community doctors with a less formal relationship to the hospital, the health system must act with evenhandedness and transparency to the fullest extent allowed by law. (Although state and federal laws do not prohibit hospitals from supporting independent physicians financially [see chapters 2 and 12], the limitations they place on such support is significant.) Hospital leaders must clearly convey a willingness to do whatever is permissible for all physicians whose practices support the hospital's mission. For example, hospitals may want to consider publicizing new employed and independent physicians with equal fanfare, even though they are not able to offer equal financial support to the independent physicians. More on this topic is presented in Chapter 13.

CAREFUL PRACTICE ACQUISITION

The first decision hospital leaders need to make when contemplating the purchase of an existing practice is about "fit." Have the physicians involved in the practice been solid citizens of the medical community? Are they productive? Are their values compatible with those of the institution? Are they mature and self-confident enough to adjust to the loss of control they will experience as an employee? Does the hospital consider their practice area important enough to the hospital's strategic direction to warrant the expenditure of energy and resources necessary to acquire it? While hospital leaders may be tempted to acquire any practice whose members request employment, they must be selective, even if unsettling departures from the medical community may result.

This admonition becomes even more important when a hospital organizes employed physicians into a formal group.

The act of practice acquisition is critical. Expectations are set on both sides that will be difficult to change downstream. The contemporary economics of physician employment will not work if money is paid for goodwill or soft assets. Hard assets need to be purchased at fair market value, and receivables should be left with the practice owners or purchased at a discounted rate that compensates for the cost of collection and bad debt. Physicians may have unrealistic fantasies about what their practices are worth. They should be educated on market trends and realities so they do not feel insulted when they are not compensated for the intangible value they perceive in their practice.

Plans for the future need to be carefully articulated. What will stay the same? What will change? For how long is stability (e.g., same office location, same staff) guaranteed? Hospitals executives too anxious to close the deal often play down the need for inevitable changes, and later, when changes are imposed, are surprised that physicians feel profoundly betrayed. Even when a hospital is unsure about the future details of its employed physician strategy (e.g., colocation of offices or formation of a group practice), it should clearly communicate that its strategy may evolve and commit to engage in an inclusive dialogue as change begins to happen.

Along the same lines, hospitals should be clear about the policies they have adopted (e.g., conflict of interest, employment guidelines, medical record requirements) that will affect physicians and their staffs. Many physicians in private practices employ family members or have long-tenured employees who may not meet the qualifications required by the hospital's personnel policies. The impact of these policies needs to be anticipated, explained, and addressed before the practice is acquired.

Finally, hospitals need to spell out their expectations for physician performance in several areas: productivity; peer relations; citizenship; participation in quality, safety, and service initiatives; and obligations, such as on-call coverage.

RECRUITMENT, INDUCTION, AND RETENTION

While hiring physicians who do not have existing practices bypasses the complexities of transitioning from independent practice, potential recruits still need to be carefully selected and clearly apprised of expectations. Incoming physicians inevitably need some mentoring on the rhythms of local practice, preferred referral relationships, and—to the extent they have been established—operational best practices that have become part of the hospital's employed physician model. To optimize practice patterns, skilled physician leaders need to ensure that feedback is delivered to new physicians respectfully and effectively during this orientation phase.

Long-term retention of good physicians involves regular attention to their satisfaction with practice in the community. The developmental needs and professional and personal aspirations of each physician should be clearly understood. Assessing these needs should be a regular and formal process; the satisfaction of employed practitioners should never be taken for granted. Not only will this attention buoy retention; happy employees are a major advantage in a competitive recruitment environment. Physician leadership is crucial to this process, as we will discuss in the sections that follow.

Even more important than retention of good doctors is retention of the *right* doctors. Some physicians may not be suited for employment, which may not be apparent until after they have been hired. When the employment relationship is not working satisfactorily for one or both parties, action should be taken to remediate the situation. Remediation requires a careful, point-by-point action plan. If remediation fails, the employment relationship should be terminated.

Some hospitals structure employment contracts in a way that requires physicians departing from the employed structure to leave the medical staff entirely. This setup ensures that embittered physicians do not remain and create unwarranted dissension. The hospital can always waive the requirement in order to keep physicians in the community if desired. Other hospitals do not link employment to medical staff membership to prevent alienating potential recruits. The trend is toward the first model—more rigorous contracts that allow the hospital to decide whether terminated physicians can remain and exercise privileges as members of the organized medical staff.

DEVELOPING THE NECESSARY BUSINESS SKILLS

Although hospitals are becoming increasingly dependent on ambulatory revenue streams to maintain profitability, the business of managing an ambulatory *physician* practice is different than the business of providing traditional hospital services or ambulatory ancillary services. Administrators trained to manage the complexities of care delivery in a hospital setting often fail when assigned to oversee the business needs generated by hospital-employed physicians. For example, the processes of coding, billing, and collecting will be different than the hospital's traditional processes for these functions, and hospital-based systems will likely be unable to accommodate the needs of physician ambulatory practice. New systems need to be built and supported by dedicated staff, or appropriate vendor relationships need to be established. Contracts with payers will need to be negotiated to include the gamut of physician procedure codes, and these negotiations will need to be informed by a nuanced understanding of how physicians in outpatient practice maximize income. Protocols and systems for collecting copayments will need to be established at every site of service. This issue is becoming increasingly relevant as payers shift the financial burden of ambulatory care to their insured.

Failure to effectively manage the practices of employed physicians creates huge dissatisfaction and reinforces many doctors' perception that hospital management is incompetent. It can also diminish the compensation of employed physicians whose income is based on collected revenues. Most hospitals would be well advised to hire practice administrators with extensive experience in outpatient and physician practice management.

ALLOCATING COST AND INCOME

The process of setting up business operations for employed physicians involves decisions that will have enormous influence on the economic viability of the employed physician model. For instance, in negotiating payer contracts, will the hospital accept smaller payments for ambulatory physician codes as a negotiating ploy to protect profitable hospital codes? If so, will it adjust budget targets for physicians accordingly? Similarly, will accounting for the group practice focus on the actual overhead of employed physicians, or will inpatient costs be shifted to the group? These decisions have important ramifications on budget setting and the calculation of physician compensation.

Hospitals also would be wise to calculate the downstream revenue attributable to employed physicians (including admissions, procedures, and diagnostic tests). An accurate picture of the economic impact of physician employment cannot be developed without consideration of these factors. For employed physicians, to be told they "lose money for the hospital" or are not efficient practitioners is demeaning when they clearly see that this characterization is a result of the hospital's accounting methodology. Feedback to employed physicians on the economics of their practice should derive from expectations set through dialogue and comparison to market benchmarks and should focus on issues that can be influenced by physician initiative.

INFRASTRUCTURE

How much space does each physician need? How should the space be configured? The answers to these questions will vary by specialty. Physicians' offices also need a variety of supplies, an approval process for minor equipment, and a streamlined restocking process not subject to the typical bureaucracy involved in requesting items from inpatient-based "central supply."

Most physicians expect they will have some "ownership" of their practice environment (in the psychological, not legal, sense), especially previously independent physicians who enter employment relationships. Hospitals need to be sensitive to these issues when they allocate and manage space. At the same time, they need to utilize space in a way that maximizes efficiency. Physicians are often colocated in large practice units unless there are strategic reasons to spread physicians throughout the marketplace. Colocation is covered extensively in a later chapter, where we elaborate on the group practice model.

Tending to the information technology needs of employed physicians is critically important. Many hospitals do not have information systems with strong modules for ambulatory practice. Hospitals need to create an entire strategy for an ambulatory electronic medical record, considering both the clinical and billing capacities of possible systems, the integration of these systems with inpatient systems, and integration across other key stakeholder populations (a local physician–hospital organization, for instance).

In all these matters, collaboration between employed physicians, practice managers, and physician leaders is essential to successful physician employment.

PRACTICE MANAGEMENT SKILLS

Practice management responsibilities include running the office on a day-to-day basis (including personnel management), designing new approaches to patient flow and care coordination, and performing specialized functions such as business development and marketing.

As healthcare migrates from a "cottage industry" to a more complex endeavor, "appropriate standardization" of ambulatory practice is becoming more necessary. Yet physicians typically resist standardization, making the process enormously challenging. At each employed physician site, a balance must be maintained between the gains of centralization/standardization and physicians' personal tastes and styles. Ambulatory physician offices operate differently than most hospital departments. Each office needs to be responsive to the particulars of the clinical specialty and the pace and tempo of its physicians.

In general, office managers of physician practices should not be accountable to managers of hospital service lines. The size of the management team for hospital affiliated physician practices needs to be established on the basis of the number of physicians and the mix of specialties composing the physician group. Reception and scheduling, clinical support, and billing and collections must also be competently performed. Most offices differentiate the responsibilities of front office staff and physician support staff (i.e., nurses and medical assistants). Office managers need to be able to supervise both sets of tasks and both pools of personnel.

The office manager's job does not stop there. Each setting requires a responsible manager able to tolerate the inevitable tension identified earlier between the need for standardization/centralization and the need for office-by-office variation. Managers also need a level of maturity and comfort balancing inevitable tension between the expectations "their" physicians have of them and the expectations the health system has for practice performance.

The office manager at each practice site needs to engage employed physicians and staff in appropriate efforts to improve office processes—from charge capture and throughput to patient education and clinical consistency. The long-term viability of the employed physician enterprise depends on this attention to the ongoing improvement of practice operations.

Finally, marketing and business development need to be undertaken in a way that extends the brand of the hospital or health system through its affiliated physicians. Physicians need to be taught how to reach out to the public, and physician offices need to be organized, decorated, and marketed in a way that clearly distinguishes them as components of an inclusive and organized system of care. When the hospital assimilates a well-recognized community practice, a clear transition plan should be created to merge the identities of both groups.

PHYSICIAN LEADERSHIP

Physician leadership emerges as a common denominator of successful care delivery enterprises. We devote an entire chapter to this matter later, where we elaborate on the factors that contribute to physician group success. Even in the absence of a group model, physician leadership is essential to successful physician employment.

The history of hospital–physician relationships and the external pressures on both parties have engendered a backlog of mistrust in many professional communities. The fact that physicians are seeking employment does not imply that suddenly all is well. Physicians often embrace employment for all of the reasons described in Chapter 3 but nonetheless enter the employment relationship with significant skepticism.

For employed physicians to feel understood by "the suits," they need to have confidence that one of their own is sitting at the table when operational issues are being discussed. Further, when it comes to accepting direction, feedback, and corrective action, physicians are more likely to respond to another physician who has "walked the walk" of clinical practice.

Physician leaders also serve as models of expected behavior—from timeliness and civility to partnership with nonphysician executives. Hospital-based physician leaders must be fully integrated with senior management, be seen as peers by the management team, and be comfortable partnering as equals with nonclinical executives—without apology and without shedding their physician identity.

The cultivation of effective physician leaders is difficult. The necessary skills are not taught in traditional medical training, nor do standard supplemental educational tracks (e.g., business courses for physicians) always provide what is promised. Through careful selection and mentoring, a pipeline of future leaders can, and should, be continuously developed.

Whether physician leaders need to remain in practice "to stay in touch" and maintain credibility is a source of great discussion in the medical community. While an understanding of practice stresses is easier to assert if one continues to do clinical work, we do not see continued practice as an absolute prerequisite for physician leaders. However, physician leaders who no longer see patients do need to have a thorough background in clinical care, remain visible in clinical environments, and be comfortable referencing their long history "in the trenches" to challenge any contention that they have gone over to the "dark side" (i.e., administration). Ultimately, the physician leader's confidence and his or her demonstrated credibility induces acceptance by peer physicians.

EXPECTATIONS AND ACCOUNTABILITY

Hospitals often hire physicians without articulating expectations or, more often, without stating expectations beyond adherence to a clinical schedule. Instead, as previously described, physicians are commonly recruited with a tacit promise that nothing about their practice will have to change. These approaches spell disaster and stem from an uncertainty about what expectations to articulate and how to express them. Hospital leaders often naively and erroneously assume that details of the employment relationship are obvious to physicians or that employment will have no effect on productive patterns of behavior well established in independent practice.

On the contrary, most physicians do not understand the unwritten nuances of employment, and physicians who have been in private practice are at risk of "relaxing into employment." Freed from the need to impose demands on themselves and absent clear expectations from others, they may begin to coast and develop feelings of entitlement.

To avoid these minefields, expectations regarding productivity, citizenship, behavior, and other institutional goals must be clearly articulated and reinforced through regular, objective performance feedback so physicians remain mindful of them.

We are frequently asked to help hospital leaders deal with physicians whom they deem "difficult." We often find out these physicians were never clearly told what was expected of them, had no help in meeting those expectations, and had received no feedback that might allow self-correction. In these circumstances, while the doctor in question may be problematic, the responsibility for the problem is usually shared by many. Such situations prove the adage that "you get the behavior you tolerate."

Regular performance evaluations tied to explicit metrics in all major areas of activity are essential to successful employment. Here again, physician leadership is essential; physician leaders are responsible for conducting a performance review process that respects the professional status and autonomy of physicians. The most successful reviews rigorously compare performance against expectations but also involve a degree of mutuality—that is, in addition to a conversation about institutional expectations, a dialogue about the physician's needs and concerns also needs to take place, beginning with the question: "How is the employment relationship working for you, Dr. [Smith], and how can we meet your needs/expectations while you meet ours?"

PART II

CHAPTER 5

From "Employed Physicians" to an "Employed Physician Group": The Critical Differences

THERE ARE SIGNIFICANT ADVANTAGES to forging employed physicians into an integrated group practice. Before a health system moves forward with a group practice development strategy, numerous factors must be considered. This chapter will provide markers of success that hospitals can use to gauge their progress toward formation of a successful, integrated group.

EMPLOYED PHYSICIANS WITHOUT AN INTEGRATED GROUP

Hospital employment of physicians is a microcosm of the American healthcare system, which has always struggled to deliver clinical services coherently. Hospitals across the United States are employing physicians in increasing numbers, but these physicians are "organized" in many small provider groups (individual practice sites and disconnected practitioners), typically as part of specialty silos. Physicians in these provider groups often practice in sites that are geographically and operationally separated from one another, which can create barriers for patients and defeat efforts at operational efficiency.

Care needs to be coordinated between primary care doctors, specialists, ancillary services, pharmacies, nursing homes, emergency centers, and hospitals, yet these organizations do not share a common infrastructure. The number of practitioners who treat patients across multiple organizational lines can be quite large, and the Babel that often ensues is not conducive to quality medical care, let alone its efficient delivery.

Despite being employed, most physicians who work for hospitals believe that autonomy is a professional right to be protected at all costs. In fact, most are assured early in the negotiation for acquisition of their services that "nothing in your practice will have to change." They feel entitled to deliver care in the manner they personally believe is best and dismiss the importance of reaching collective decisions with their peers or employing best practices or standardized protocols.

Leadership structures for hospital-employed physicians vary from one organization to another. In many cases, the office staff members who serve the employed doctors answer to a member of the hospital executive team, but to whom the physicians themselves report is often unclear. Frequently a medical director, VPMA, or CMO is given the administrative role to serve as *liaison* between the doctors and the hospital executive suite. This physician executive may be responsible for managing ten physicians or hundreds, without any clear mandate or authority.

In contrast to the layers of management dedicated to the administration of other hospital employees (e.g., nurses, techs, housekeepers, security personnel), infrastructure devoted to the management of employed physicians is usually insubstantial. Few businesses in America would consider deploying a critical workforce with such minimal supervision. Employed physicians are often unclear about whom they are accountable to, and the managerial oversight and support physicians receive are inadequate.

Physician practices acquired by a hospital often are allowed to maintain their existing informatics technology, slowing the shift to common electronic medical records and uniform data collection.

Similarly, they may maintain previous office staff, office policies and reporting structures, practice protocols, and equipment sources. As a result, a hospital that is building a cohort of employed doctors may be securing a portion of its critical physician workforce, but it is not necessarily moving toward a more efficient and effective delivery *system*. Migrating these employed doctors toward a true integrated group practice is the key to realizing the advantages of coordinated care.

STRENGTHS OF THE INTEGRATED GROUP PRACTICE MODEL

Some of the most successful and prestigious medical organizations in the nation are large group practices or clinics (see Exhibit 5.1). In many of these organizations, physician leadership nurtured within the group practice provides critical guidance to the entire health system. Mayo Clinic, for example, is world renowned for its quality of care and patient service. It is a center of high-tech,

---

Exhibit 5.1 A Sample of Prestigious Medical Groups

Mayo Clinic, MN
Ochsner Clinic, LA
Cleveland Clinic, OH
Geisinger Health System, PA
Scott & White Clinic, TX
Lahey Clinic, MA
Henry Ford Health System, MI
Permanente Medical Group, CA
Aurora Health, WI
Carle Clinic, IL
Guthrie Clinic, PA and NY
Billings Clinic, MT
Gundersen Clinic, WI, MN, and IA

---

leading-edge medicine, yet it has some of the lowest costs for care in the nation. Its physicians, considered among the best in their fields, participate in a culture of teamwork that involves clinic staff at all levels. Mayo Clinic is an enormous, complex organization, yet it functions with great efficiency and consistently delivers high value to those paying for care. In this age of dispirited clinicians, morale is reportedly high among its medical staff members.

Is Mayo's success an aberration? Or do group practices have inherent advantages that make them a preferred model for delivering high-quality, efficient, innovative, and cost-effective care to the great satisfaction of patients and providers?

The nation's leading group practices have grown organically from a small nucleus of colleagues who wanted to experiment with a different approach to the practice of medicine. Often they did so against considerable peer disapproval (see Exhibit 5.2). The values that set them apart and underscored their successes have had a chance to sink into the culture of their organizations for many decades.

What makes large group practices so effective and such a foundational element in health systems that seek greater integration and better performance? Fundamentally, true group practices have a value structure that emphasizes involvement, peer leadership, and decision making with the best interests of the entire organization in mind. This combination involves compromise on two levels—

Exhibit 5.2 The Ochsner Story: 30 Pieces of Silver

The Ochsner Clinic in New Orleans (now the Ochsner Health System) was founded in 1942 by five committed physicians considered leaders in their medical community. Their medical colleagues felt betrayed by the prospect of a new model of care. Each of the five founders received an anonymous "gift" recalling that which Judas accepted: small leather pouches containing 30 dimes (pure silver at the time). Each pouch contained a typewritten note: "To help pay for your clinic...from the physicians, surgeons, and dentists of New Orleans."

---

between individual and collective desires, and between standardized and individualized practices. The resulting value structure is a marked departure from that which doctors bring to most healthcare organizations. When this structure is married to a strong work ethic and sophisticated business operations, the foundation for success is locked in place.

What these group practices achieve is no less than a refashioning of the historic "culture of the expert" inculcated into doctors through the rigors of their lengthy medical education. In the culture of the expert, the doctor is accountable for all that happens. Physicians are taught to trust no one—to always check the patient, X-rays, lab tests, and studies to ensure nothing has been overlooked or reported incorrectly. They are taught to act decisively—there is no time for group process when patients need immediate care and the doctor in charge is accountable for everything. And they are taught to be suspicious of administrators, who, lacking medical degrees, are imagined to have nothing to contribute to clinical decisions, and too often are thought to put the needs of the institution before those of the patient.

The culture of the expert insists that doctors are the patient's advocates before they are patients' advocates. In this culture, a good doctor puts the apostrophe before the *s*, whereas administrators place the apostrophe after it. Doctors are taught to concentrate on the trees, not the forest. The culture of the expert also encourages doctors to put their own needs before the needs of other healthcare providers. The consequence is physician-centric care that engenders patient and staff dissatisfaction. This culture may have been appropriate when modern medicine was coming of age in the twentieth century, but it is not suited to care delivery in complex health systems facing myriad organizational challenges.

Transforming a long-engrained practice culture is a daunting task. Many hospitals and health systems are struggling to inculcate a stronger atmosphere of teamwork and greater attention to quality. Most are experiencing only minimal success because physician interests are not adequately aligned with hospital interests. Physician employment modestly increases alignment, but hospital administrators cannot simply require physicians to change their practice culture, even when the doctors work under an employment agreement. Sustained initiative by physician leaders, legitimized and accepted by their professional peers, is necessary to transform culture.

Successful group practices are characterized by their ability to move past the culture of the expert and create a different work climate. These practices pride themselves on teamwork and collaboration, value a systems approach to care, and see physicians and administrators as colleagues who can achieve more when they work in concert. They support efforts to standardize care around best practices and are more likely to be interested in the health of their communities and not just their patients. They eschew historic peer review practices of "shame and blame," and their member physicians work to improve each other's clinical practice through supportive, collegial efforts. Overall, they embrace a culture more responsive to the demands of patients, employers, politicians, payers, and the many external parties clamoring for a better care delivery system.

Because group practice culture values coordination, teamwork, and collaboration, these organizations are usually early adopters of information technology. Electronic medical records are essential to successful integration of care delivery across multiple providers and multiple sites. Group practices historically have been quick to recognize the necessity of having computerized records that can be easily shared between providers and across geographic locations. These groups are also more likely to have the financial resources to invest in these tools, in contrast to physicians in small practices who have enormous difficulty generating the dollars necessary to purchase a complex technological infrastructure. Full integration within complex health systems simply cannot be completed without a backbone of electronic health records.

Successful group practices are better able to address the multiple needs of their patients because they are organized to attend to numerous clinical issues simultaneously, and in a coordinated way. In contrast, for a physician in solo practice, the scope of elements that must be coordinated to help patients navigate today's healthcare world is overwhelming. The small practice physician has neither the time nor staff to do this work, and this endeavor is not cost-effective when undertaken alone.

Mayo Clinic and its counterparts are excellent examples of organizations that can bring substantial resources to bear on servicing the patient (Beery and Seltman 2008). Multiple specialists, linked by a common electronic health record, gather around the patient, whatever the patient's needs. Keeping the patient as the central focus of the care delivery process has been part of Mayo's organizational culture since the Mayo brothers established their clinic. As patients become more knowledgeable and more demanding consumers of healthcare, they will be drawn to large group practices that are highly responsive to their desires for convenience and seamless coordination. Patients describe their experiences with well-functioning groups as being "held"; whatever the medical issue, a team member is ready to respond.

Group practices value teamwork and assert that value forcefully. Physicians who are extremely independent in their work habits, who value autonomy above all else, and who don't work well with staff fit poorly in group practices. These physicians usually aren't hired into successful group practices. When they are hired, their employment with the practice usually doesn't last. Integrated multispecialty practices commit to teamwork as a core cultural value and look for every occasion to reinforce it. Methods of reinforcement range from setting clear expectations for collaboration and cooperation to evaluating the manifestation of these attributes in physician members of the group and using the resulting data in compensation and advancement formulas.

Group practices situated within an integrated delivery system have yet another powerful advantage. Because of their control over a broad range of resources, financial stability, strong leadership, and history of collaboration and teamwork, they tend to be innovative. In these turbulent times, a future of constant change in healthcare is a certainty. The nature of that change is less clear. Many healthcare organizations are not well positioned to adapt quickly to unanticipated changes. For example, small private physician practices have been blindsided by the changing expectations of their newest young colleagues. They face huge recruitment challenges as the physician shortage worsens and younger physicians migrate toward employment by large, stable organizations. Integrated delivery systems with strong group practices can tap the creativity and energy of physician leaders to quickly respond to changing patient expectations, new models of reimbursement, the growth of regulatory constraints, new "disruptive" technologies, demands for workflow redesign, and whatever else the future has in store. Geisinger's decision to "warranty" open heart surgery is a perfect example of this ability to respond. See Exhibit 5.3 below.

A final advantage of large integrated group practices is their ability to implement the patient-centered medical home (PCMH)—a practice model garnering rapid support. Numerous professional groups, employers, payers, and government entities have endorsed this approach to coordinated clinical care. For instance, the National Committee for Quality Assurance has an accreditation program for group practices implementing this model. In a large national study commissioned by The Commonwealth Fund, large physician

---

Exhibit 5.3 Geisinger "Warranties" Open Heart Surgery

Healthcare systems across the country have been attacked for using opaque pricing, providing poor value, failing to follow through with treatment plans—the list goes on. Responding to these criticisms, the Geisinger Health System in Pennsylvania began to guarantee cardiac patients and payers that it would address any preventable complications that might arise as a result of heart surgery at no cost. Geisinger is confident in its ability to deliver care with minimal complications and could make this commitment to the public because of the seamless integration of physicians, hospitals, and administrative staff. All are aligned, committed, and involved—together. This example captures the essence of the group practice advantage.

---

group practices were found to be best positioned to implement this model. PCMHs not only deliver higher-quality, more coordinated, and more patient-friendly care but also realize significant financial savings (Rittenhouse et al. 2008; State of North Carolina, Office of the Governor 2007; Community Care of North Carolina 2008).

IS A MOVE TOWARD GREATER PHYSICIAN EMPLOYMENT AND HEALTH SYSTEM INTEGRATION THE RIGHT STRATEGY FOR EVERY ORGANIZATION?

Moving from a constellation of individual employed physicians to an integrated multispecialty clinic is not something that can happen overnight; it is a complex process. Before a hospital decides to embark down this path, it must assess its ability to achieve the desired end. Before committing to the development of a truly integrated group practice, a health system's senior leadership and board must consider a number of factors:

1. *Does the hospital/health system have the financial resources to form a group practice?*

   As noted in an earlier chapter, hospitals in the past often employed primary care physicians to capture the "covered lives" of managed care organizations. Today, many hospitals also employ specialists to secure their essential or more lucrative service lines. Practitioners such as neurosurgeons, cardiothoracic and general surgeons, and orthopedic and trauma specialists are often the first to be employed. These physicians are expensive to employ, and as the number of specialists on the payroll grows, securing their referral base to protect the hospital's investment becomes more important. Thus, the more specialists a hospital hires, the more it needs to simultaneously add primary care physicians to the staff. Before doing so, a hospital should make sure it has the economic strength to add all the doctors it will need to create a stable group.

Hospitals also need to assess other financial burdens. Close integration with physicians requires a serious commitment to implementing electronic medical records and other informatics technology. The quicker these tools are in place, the more attractive the group practice will be to new physicians and the more effective the practice will be in meeting health system goals. Implementation of electronic medical records is an expensive proposition requiring a longitudinal budgetary commitment over and above other integration costs. Before a board undertakes a strategic plan built around a newly developed large employed group practice, it must review the gamut of budgetary considerations.

2. *Can the hospital/health system find or make available appropriate ambulatory practice space?*

Another expensive ingredient essential to physician integration is carefully designed office space that can accommodate a multispecialty practice and provide one-stop "shopping" for patients. Consolidating acquired practices into common locations often requires creation of new office space or radical reconfiguration of existing office space and strategic redeployment of physicians to capture market share. We elaborate on this important element in Chapter 10.

3. *Should the hospital partner with another hospital or health system before moving toward greater physician integration?*

There are several reasons the hospital board may want to consider this option. If the hospital is not in a strong financial position, it may want to team up with an organization that is. As noted earlier, physician employment is an expensive endeavor. The hospital also may want to forestall direct and damaging competition with another player that is in the marketplace or looking to enter it. A hospital's battle to retain autonomy and sole control over the physicians in its region may end with a

Pyrrhic victory if it exhausts its resources in the effort. A hospital might also be located in a geographic area that does not attract physicians, even when they are offered the option of employment. If the hospital joins a system that has a strong track record of physician recruitment and employment, that system's larger group practice may be able to establish satellite physician offices in the less compelling geographic market.

4. *Will the hospital employ its entire medical staff at some point, or does it envision an integrated system that also includes physicians in private practice?*

   This decision depends on multiple factors and may change over time. As stated previously, group practice is not an appealing setting for everyone (more on this topic in chapters to come); some physicians may be valuable members of the medical community but would not work well in a group. Hospitals need to recruit selectively, which means they must be prepared to reject such applicants. Private practices provide a home for such physicians and can be aligned with the interests of the hospital even in the absence of tight integration. A mixed model (employed and private practice doctors on staff) may also allow the health system to stage the expansion of its employed medical group and spread the economic burden over a longer period, while accommodating those who prefer or are better suited for traditional practice models.

   On the other hand, if a hospital is in a competitive marketplace, it may not want to leave market share to private physicians who could be attracted to neighboring hospitals, health systems, or management companies looking to capture new market share. In addition, the quicker a hospital moves to full integration with an employed group practice, the more competitive it will be with other hospitals pursuing the same strategy.

5. *Is the hospital's administrative team capable of pulling off an integrated model?*

   Moving to a delivery system that employs its physician base is a challenging undertaking. Management teams that have been successful at running "bricks and mortar" facilities may not be up to the task of managing a complex integrated system. A willingness to frankly assess management bench strength and expand the senior leadership team as necessary is critical.

6. *Is there a sufficient level of trust between the hospital board/ management team and community doctors?*

   Trust is an essential ingredient in building any kind of tightly integrated team. A history of significant mistrust between administrators and the community's doctors will jeopardize the success of any integration effort. The hospital board may need to appoint new leaders to alleviate historical misgivings and build the tight relationships that characterize the most successful integrated delivery systems. If the board is not willing to make leadership changes, it may make the task of building an employed group more difficult; trustworthiness may need to be proven again and again.

7. *Are the board and health system management team willing to cede significant authority to physicians in the employed or affiliated group?*

   Successful group practices have strong physician leadership. Many of the most successful integrated systems in the nation are physician driven. As healthcare delivery migrates away from inpatient facilities, system leaders will lean more heavily on the skills, knowledge, and insights of physician leaders to accomplish their goals. Physician management is a fundamental, core element of powerful integrated systems, far more critical than the oversight of facilities. If this trend is threatening to the health system's top management, its board should think twice before adopting a strategy of greater physician employment and integration. At a minimum, it should be committed to allowing the employed physician group practice to exercise increasing self-governance as the group matures. (The governance activities of group practices are discussed in Chapter 7.) Once employed physicians master this critical role, the health system board's willingness to give them greater responsibility across the enterprise can transform an organization in powerful and valuable ways (see Chapter 13).

MEASURES OF SUCCESS

When a hospital employs a significant number of doctors and embraces group formation, how will it be able to track its progress toward true practice integration? An organization can use the following indicators to evaluate the development of group cohesion:

- A physician-driven governance structure for the group practice is in place.
- The physicians have an articulated, shared vision for the group practice.
- A unitary infrastructure and management framework supports all specialties and practice locations.
- The group practice management team comprises different administrators than those managing the hospital.
- The group promulgates standardized clinical approaches.
- Few referrals are made to physicians outside the group when the clinical services are available in-house.
- Physicians are compensated according to a unitary system that they manage through their governance body.
- All members of the group share a brand identity.
- Group members are able to resolve disputes among themselves internally, without requiring the intervention of hospital administrators. (An example would be a turf dispute between specialties over appropriate privileges to perform a procedure.)
- The group promotes a common culture by establishing clear expectations for physicians who join and by mentoring new physicians.
- The group maintains accountability through clear structures and processes.

- The group is able to reject for membership physicians who do not fit its culture and vision.

MOVING EMPLOYED PHYSICIANS INTO AN INTEGRATED GROUP PRACTICE: THE WORK OF IMPLEMENTATION

How does a hospital begin building an integrated multispecialty group practice? When developing a strategic plan for growing a group practice and moving to greater integration, hospitals need to set a reasonable timeline that will work in the context of a health system's community and resources. Move too slowly, and momentum and enthusiasm may be lost. Move too quickly, and physicians' innate discomfort with change may provoke resistance to the initiative.

No single formula can be applied to all institutions seeking to integrate physicians, but having a clearly constructed game plan is critical. Significant input from the practice community and hospital and system leaders should be solicited and considered when crafting this plan. It needs to envision an evolving process of integration and pay attention to the sequencing and timing of change. Steps that will bring about revolutionary change (e.g., migration to a common medical record) need to be distinguished from stages that will develop in an evolutionary way (e.g., the evolving role of the group practice governing body). As with any complex project, attention to indicators of progress (metrics and milestones) will enable real-time fine tuning.

Gathering data on the practice community will help gauge the speed with which doctors will be able to make decisions about employment options. For example, survey tools can be used to gather information on physicians' readiness to integrate more fully with the health system (see Exhibit 5.4). Health system leaders also should communicate with practice managers of larger private practices in the community and with the physicians in these groups. The practice managers may be good resources for the developing hospital group practice, or they may be a source of significant resistance when the physicians in a private group consider hospital employment.

Exhibit 5.4 Surveying the Physician Community to Assess Readiness for Integration: Sample Questions (typically answered on a scale of 1–5)

1. Do you believe that physicians in our community can work successfully in close cooperation with the senior management team of ABC Health System to achieve closer alignment of their interests?
2. Do you believe that tighter integration of community physicians with ABC Health System will lead to improved healthcare in our region?
3. To what extent do you believe that a closer integration of physician practices and health system services would improve the following?
   a. Patient satisfaction
   b. Coordination of care
   c. Quality and patient safety
   d. Physician morale and satisfaction in practice
   e. Ability to recruit new clinical practitioners to the community
   f. Flow of clinical information across providers
   g. Cost-effectiveness of care
   h. Responsiveness of patient care services
   i. Satisfaction of physician office staff
   j. Satisfaction of health system staff
   k. Reputation of healthcare in the community
   l. Ability to capture increased revenue under pay-for-performance formulas
   m. Leverage with payers to achieve reimbursement schedules
   n. Retention of current community practitioners
4. Do you believe development of a hospital-owned physician group practice will reduce out-migration of patients seeking care?
5. Do you believe that geographic consolidation of physician practices in multispecialty offices is a desirable goal?
6. What are your three greatest concerns about future integration of ABC Health System and community physicians?

(Continued on following page)

7. What do you see as the three greatest advantages that would result from further integration of ABC Health System with its community physicians?
8. Please describe what you believe would be the greatest obstacle to greater integration between community physicians and ABC Health System.

Careful consideration should be given to the compensation model that will be offered to doctors when they join. Initially, this model will need to be fairly straightforward so that doctors clearly understand what the transition to employment will mean for them financially. However, with time, control over the model will need to be given to the physicians' governing body so it can be refined to support and reward the values of the group, reflect changing market realities, and support the goals of the integrated system.

Many hospitals will not have the internal resources or experience needed to craft a solid tactical plan for moving to an integrated model. In such cases, the hospital should consult external experts who have worked in the delicate interface between doctors and hospitals. These professionals can assess the medical community's readiness to embrace a physician integration strategy and give an honest appraisal of whether the requisite trust exists for an effective collaboration. If they find the hospital is in a good position to move forward, they can propose appropriate integration models and design financial models of the various options. In addition, they can design an initial compensation model for physicians considering employment that is clear and easy to evaluate.

CONCLUSION

The decision to commit to a strategy of integration with an emerging physician group practice is never simple and never easy. The ability of a health system to successfully support such a strategy may be uncertain, but the worthiness of the goal is becoming increasingly clear. In 2001 the Institute of Medicine (IOM) issued a landmark report, *Crossing the Quality Chasm*, to provide direction for our dysfunctional American healthcare system. This report argued that healthcare should be safe, effective, patient-centered, timely, efficient, and equitable. Only successful integrated health systems anchored by strong multidisciplinary physician groups demonstrate the ability to achieve IOM's goals. From this perspective, health systems and physicians must seriously consider whether they can afford *not* to pursue greater integration through the model of group practice formation.

CHAPTER 6

Group Practice Evolution: The Path of Change

FORGING A HIGH-FUNCTIONING, integrated group requires commitment, perseverance, and considerable skill. A detailed strategic plan will help health systems avoid the pitfalls that can waylay efforts at group practice development. This strategy needs to articulate the envisioned end state of functional integration and drive a series of operational steps that must be taken to make that vision a reality. In this chapter, we will outline those steps.

ENSURING INSTITUTIONAL COMMITMENT; ENGAGING THE EXECUTIVE TEAM

In most cases, health systems cannot employ a significant number of physicians or form group practices without the support of top leadership. Health system boards rarely endorse their organizations' strategy for physician employment if their chief executive officer does not support the initiative.

Convincing health system executives and managers to support a strategy for group practice formation may be a daunting task. Physicians merging into an integrated group practice usually push for strong self-governance and significant control over their affairs. Some health systems even articulate an explicit long-term strategy to develop into physician-led organizations. In such cases, members of the executive team may feel threatened. Administrators often perceive physicians as unqualified for organizational leadership roles. When asked to characterize physicians, many executives describe them as anarchic and incapable of working on a team or in a bureaucracy, overly reactive, and self-serving. They are inclined to assert that physicians are poor planners, make rash decisions, and do not share the same sense of loyalty to the institution.

Members of the "C-suite" (e.g., chief executive, operating, financial, nursing, and medical officers) are generally experienced at running the inpatient programs of a hospital or health system. They may be affronted by the suggestion that physicians can become better suited to drive the enterprise and that administration will become less about facilities management and more about achieving broad health agendas. They may also be dismayed to see the diversion of system resources from their own areas of control to the expensive undertaking of establishing an integrated multispecialty group practice.

Reluctant or resistant executives will impede the movement toward greater physician–hospital integration if they cannot be persuaded that the strategy is sound. In most cases, the CEO will have to garner the support of his or her leadership team through a variety of tactics.

The first of these tactics is education. Rationale for integration with physicians can be evidenced through the literature, presentations by outside consultants, and field trips to successful models. Visits to other organizations can be especially helpful, where executives can hear from colleagues how their organizations have been improved by greater integration with physicians. Incumbent executives can learn how increased physician alignment within a health system drives greater physician engagement in projects important to senior administrators. To debrief the experience, members of the top management team should engage in a discussion in which each participant voices his or her opinions and perceptions. Where appropriate, the CEO can follow up with one-on-one conversations.

Second, the CEO needs to assign responsibility for group development to one member of the hospital's senior management team. While this executive may rely on others to address operational needs, he or she should have sufficient seniority and experience to deal with delicate, complex issues and engage in potentially high-risk/high-gain negotiations with key physicians.

Third, the hospital or system board should express to the management team that it has embraced the physician group practice strategy and is irrevocably committed to its success—and reaffirm this support whenever it has the opportunity. Repeated declarations of institutional commitment will reassure new physicians that the hospital is serious about their future success, as well as clarify the hospital's mission to the rest of its community.

Finally, links should be made between every executive's portfolio of responsibilities and the plans for group formation. Such accountability makes success a collective responsibility. As mentioned earlier, most of the executive team will express support for a physician integration strategy once they understand how it can drive operational success and the board has endorsed it. Those who do so with half-hearted enthusiasm are likely to gain confidence in the initiative over time. Executives who cling to former management models and refuse to buy in to the approach should be advised that they will not be a good fit for the organization over the long term, and transition planning for a move to a more appropriate venue should ensue.

Emerging physician leaders in the group practice will need coaching as well. They need to enter the management structure with an appreciation for the skills of nonphysician executives and demonstrate an ability to partner around mutual goals. Operational authority can be shared with emerging physician leaders only to the extent that these leaders develop collaborative skills.

EXTENDING INSTITUTIONAL COMMITMENT THROUGH THE LEADERSHIP RANKS

Most knowledgeable hospital executive teams quickly come to understand the market dynamics that make a physician integration strategy essential and the value of developing a hospital-owned physician group practice. Middle management, however, is often not so easy to convince.

Middle managers usually defend their turf. Having been through repeated hospital cost-saving initiatives, they are sensitized to system activities that may divert dollars from their areas of responsibility. Also, these managers are adept at working within a bureaucratic hierarchy that shields them against the vagaries of the doctors with whom they interact. For many midlevel hospital administrators, the typical physician is difficult to manage and is someone from whom they must protect their established work routines and staff. A health system vision that employs physicians and increasingly involves them in the control of day-to-day affairs can be a frightening prospect to middle management. The result may be passive-aggressive behavior that undermines the development of doctor–administrator teams and the collaboration that must take place for a hospital to capture the full value of physician integration.

To combat this resistance, all members of the hospital's management team should be made to feel a part of the integration initiative. Regular meetings should be held with middle managers to educate them on the strategy and keep them informed about the initiative's progress. These sessions can be used to recount success stories of physician–manager collaboration. Midlevel administrators from well-functioning integrated delivery systems can be invited to share their experiences and relate how they overcame challenges along the way. Dedicating at least half a day each quarter to such meetings can significantly undercut the group's inherent resistance to change. Such meetings are a venue for engaging these critical health system leaders in the organization's affiliated-group strategy.

This time can also be used to clarify the message they should pass on to the rest of the staff. As physicians become more involved in the system, they will play an increasing role in redesigning traditional hospital workflow. The managers of frontline hospital staff will need to explain and support the changes that occur and help their reports acquire the skills they need to engage with their physician partners constructively.

The next step in enlisting support involves outreach to the public. The board should endorse a communication initiative that explains to the community why it will be well-served by the hospital's employment of physicians. The public needs to understand that this development will help control costs and provide a more stable cohort of doctors, a higher level of responsiveness to patients and their families, and seamless, higher-quality care. When they take this position publically, the board and health system leaders demonstrate unequivocal commitment to the creation of a group practice comprising employed physicians.

ESTABLISH A GOVERNING BODY FOR THE PHYSICIAN GROUP

The greatest anxiety physicians have about moving from private practice to hospital employment concerns loss of autonomy. To reassure physicians that they will be able to exercise some self-direction and participate in critical decision making, a mechanism for physician governance should be established early in the development of a hospital-owned group practice.

First, the senior administrator responsible for the emerging group should, after discussion with key physicians, appoint an interim board or executive committee and, in concert with an elected chair of that body, guide the board through the early stages of its work. The first few meetings of this group should be devoted to understanding the group practice model, exploring the case for group practice formation, and embracing the task of leading the group forward.

Depending on the number of physicians who will compose the initial group, the interim board may include as few as 5 members or as many as 15. Boards of more than 15 members are generally unwieldy; appointment of 7 to 12 members is usually optimal. The interim board should include physicians who represent the breadth of the group in terms of both clinical services and geography. Key hospital executives charged with driving and supporting group formation should attend board meetings but not be eligible to vote on board actions.

The interim board's job is to communicate with the employed physician community. It explains upcoming changes, addresses concerns, and fosters enthusiasm about the plan for group formation (or at least openness to group formation). Beyond learning, committing to the group practice vision, and reaching out, the interim board is responsible for chartering several key committees. These committees should be led by members of the interim board and supported by hospital staff. They should also include group physicians who are not members of the interim board but wish to be involved in the group practice's development.

Initiate a Group of Critical Board Committees

Compensation, culture, quality, and operations are topics that warrant early attention. Board committees commit to a steep learning curve on behalf of the interim board and lead deliberations related to each topic. If the hospital is aggressively growing its community of employed physicians, it may also need to charter a recruitment committee. As we will describe at greater length in Chapter 7, these committees recommend paths of action to the board but do not have decision-making power.

- *Compensation committee*: Compensation will likely be inconsistent among the employed physicians who compose the initial practice group. Deals will have been made individually with these physicians, sometimes negotiated by different hospital executives and often based on varying business models and institutional needs.

Developing a consistent approach to compensation that is easy to understand, equitable, and as simple as possible will be a critical task during the group's first years. To guide the development of a uniform scheme, the compensation committee needs to learn how established groups approach payment (see Chapter 10), determine appropriate measures of productivity, and decide on other areas of performance for which physicians will be eligible for financial rewards.

- *Culture committee*: One of the great challenges in launching a group practice is energizing a commitment to mutually accepted values and shared behavioral expectations. The successful groups described in previous chapters have had the advantage of being able to develop norms gradually, over decades. Without institutional memory and a cadre of seasoned group members to model and enforce norms, fledgling group practices have to rely on carefully focused work to establish clear group expectations. Often the culture committee develops these expectations into a statement of principles or code of conduct, which is then presented to the board for discussion and adoption.

- *Quality committee*: One of the compelling arguments for group formation is that integration and collaboration will result in improved outcomes. These improved outcomes will instill a sense of pride in the group and justify charging payers premium rates. For these reasons, focus should be placed on quality expectations in the formative months of the group practice. The quality committee's job is to galvanize the group's nascent leaders into prioritizing the development of quality targets and adopting methodologies for meeting those targets.

- *Operations committee*: If attention to quality can be described as *effectiveness,* then attention to operations can be referred to as *efficiency*. An increase in both effectiveness and efficiency translates into value of profound proportions. The first step of the operations committee's job is studying efficiency among the group's providers and offices and identifying patterns of variation. Energy can then be devoted to multiple objectives, including

- appropriate consolidation of practices,
- appropriate standardization of practices,
- development of a shared information platform,
- increased effectiveness of inpatient operations,
- smoother inpatient/outpatient transitions,
- marketing and branding initiatives, and
- minimization of referral leakage outside the group.

Attention to these objectives needs to be prioritized according to the circumstances of each group. While most of the responsibility for operational improvements defaults to the group's nonphysician staff, the involvement of physicians in initial planning and review is critical. We will discuss the keys to operational success in detail in chapters 10 and 11. Here, we simply want to stress the need to plan for operational success in the early stages of group formation.

Because ultimate oversight of the employed group's financial performance takes place at the hospital or system level, many employed groups do not have a separate finance committee and delegate financial review to the compensation or operations committee. Other groups create finance committees in their early stages to educate physicians about the financial repercussions of practice patterns, review the practice's financial performance, and propose ways to increase profitability.

EMPLOY A PHYSICIAN EXECUTIVE

While the board determines group policy, board members have "day jobs" as practitioners. They come together to lend their wisdom and perspective to major decisions but do not necessarily have the time, inclination, or skills to execute the group's initiatives. For this reason, groups of substantial size employ a physician executive to oversee the practice's activities. In freestanding groups, this person is often appointed as group CEO. A team of subordinate executives, including a chief medical officer (CMO), is also usually appointed. In hospital-employed groups, ultimate authority rests with a member of the hospital or system executive team, typically the hospital vice president of medical affairs (VPMA) or health system CMO, for whom group supervision is only one task in a portfolio of other duties.

In either case, the complexities of managing and building the group practice require the ongoing attention of an additional experienced physician executive. This individual, commonly called the group CMO or medical director, partners with a nonphysician administrator to run the group's operations. In smaller groups, this position may be part time, but as groups grow to include 50 or more providers, the need for a full-time medical director becomes increasingly urgent.

This individual is responsible for translating hospital and board priorities into operational terms, clarifying expectations, providing performance feedback to group members, and leading change initiatives. He or she mentors emerging physician leaders as they become oriented to new roles. This person is also indispensible in managing the sensitive relationships among the physicians and practices that have been merged into the group.

In most cases, incumbent VPMAs and hospital/system CMOs, already charged with more than they can handle, cannot stretch to provide this operational leadership in an emerging group. Time and again, however, hospital management teams make the mistake of piling even more responsibilities on incumbents rather than investing resources in creating a new position. Many would agree that managing doctors is more demanding than managing the average hospital staff employee. Hospitals typically employ a significant number of managers per hundred employees but only one VPMA or CMO to manage hundreds of physicians. Hospitals building an employed group medical practice are advised not to shortchange their investment in experienced physician leadership and should recruit a medical director with group practice management experience if possible.

Initially, the group practice medical director should have a dual reporting relationship to the responsible health system executive and to the group practice board. However, the group practice governing body should have final say over the hiring and firing of a practice medical director. In this way there will be clarity about the medical director's accountability to the group.

The group practice medical director should have a comprehensive job description that creates clear formal authority to make decisions that implement the health system's strategy and reflect the board's policies, thereby bringing policy to life within the group practice. This job description should be reviewed and approved by the governing body. It should clearly identify the medical director's responsibilities and his or her authority to act on behalf of the practice board and the health system. This role is different than the traditional hospital VPMA role, which is usually advisory in nature. The VPMA serves as a liaison between the hospital and doctors but rarely has the authority to take direct action. A medical director limited to an advisory role cannot accomplish the volume of work required to create a powerful group practice.

Instead of using the popularity-based voting process typically used to appoint medical staff, physicians should use a search and interview approach to select the medical director. This method removes some of the politics from the process and focuses the physicians' attention on the competencies necessary for success in the job.

There is a common belief that, for political reasons, most physician communities prefer to appoint a medical director who is already an employed member of the group. This assumption is logical from the viewpoint that appointment of an incumbent physician—particularly a popular one—would be less disruptive to group continuity and soften the impact of change. "Staying in the family" is risky, however, unless the physician

1. has administrative leadership experience,

2. has demonstrated an aptitude for dealing with complex and conflicted situations, and
3. is genuinely open to coaching from external advisors.

To be effective in the role, an incumbent medical director must have these three attributes.

BUILD AN EXPERIENCED PRACTICE MANAGEMENT TEAM

Repurposing hospital managers as group administrative staff is usually a mistake. Many of the group's physicians will have worked closely with their own support staff in independent practice. They will quickly recognize inexperience or ineptitude. Such repurposing was prevalent during the first wave of practice acquisition and physician employment in the 1990s. The use of weak practice management staff led to poor financial results and incurred the anger and dismay of physicians. Hospitals lost precious credibility by failing to demonstrate practice management competency.

Unless one of the group's constituent practices has a star manager with enormous potential, an experienced practice director should be recruited to oversee day-to-day operations. The interim board should be involved in screening candidates for this job, but the practice director should report directly to the senior executive responsible for the group's success.

This individual has the challenging job of building a unified team from the workforces of each physician's office staff (see Chapter 10). The practice director needs to establish clear personnel policies (most often identical to those of the hospital) and a consistent process for assessing the needs of each office and the talents and potential of current practice staff. He or she needs to lay out a clear plan for centralizing administrative functions (e.g., billing), decentralizing office management, and developing support staff flexibility and cross-coverage capacities.

The group also needs the guidance of a dedicated finance director and the support of other hospital departments (e.g., marketing, human resources, facilities management, information technology). The need for personnel fully dedicated to these ancillary functions depends on group size and local conditions.

COMMUNICATION AND MEMBER ENGAGEMENT

As the activities described above take place, usually over 12 to 18 months, the interim board should be in constant contact with the employed physicians who constitute the group. The medical director and practice director similarly have the ongoing tasks of building support for the group and addressing concerns. The board committees' work needs to be shared and discussed with group members so they can provide input and accept emerging policies (including new approaches to compensation).

The interim board needs to develop policies dictating the composition of the formal board and establish a nominating and election process. At the group's first election, the interim board stands down in favor of the new, formal board. We will describe in Chapter 7 the way an ad hoc nominating committee can facilitate the selection of board members.

The induction of the first formal board is an important milestone in the development of the new group and should be celebrated with fanfare, including a formal blessing of the hospital or system board and CEO.

CONCLUSION

The first year of a hospital affiliated group practice's development is a critical time. Letting the group grow haphazardly can be a fatal early misstep. Careful attention to the developmental steps outlined in this chapter and summarized in Exhibit 6.1 is a foundation for continued growth and long-term success for the new group practice enterprise.

Exhibit 6.1 Early Steps in the Development of a Hospital-Owned Multispecialty Group Practice

- Research the process and costs of implementing an integrated group practice strategy.
- Confirm institutional commitment at the level of the health system board.
- Establish senior management's commitment to the strategy.
- Assign responsibility for group practice formation and effectiveness to one member of the senior executive team.
- Educate middle management on the initiative's vision, goals, and processes.
- Create an interim governing board for the group practice and establish its authority.
- Create governing board subcommittees to address such issues as
    - creation of a group practice identity, culture, and brand;
    - oversight of operational and financial performance;
    - promulgation of a quality/performance improvement agenda; and
    - creation of a compensation model.
- Hire a group practice medical director.
- Agree on a process for identifying potential recruits and vetting them to the practice (or designate a recruitment committee for this task).
- Establish an administrative team under the direction of an experienced group practice operations director.
- Formally launch the new structure.

CHAPTER 7

Group Practice Governance

THE CREATION, EDUCATION, AND GRADUAL EMPOWERMENT of an interim governing body are critical early steps in group practice formation. The subsequent transition from an interim board to an elected board is a seminal step in the evolution of the integrated group practice.

THE GROUP PRACTICE BOARD AND ITS RELATIONSHIP TO THE HOSPITAL OR HEALTH SYSTEM

Self-governance is one of the defining characteristics of a successful group practice. Self-governed groups face the challenge of defining a unique, collective identity; establishing a culture; and shaping the character of collective practice. The creation of an effective governance structure is an essential step in moving from a cluster of separate practices to a unitary group.

The board is responsible for articulating the group practice's guiding principles. The terms *mission* (what business are we in?), *vision* (where are we setting our sights?), and *values* (what principles guide our work?) are often used to capture these overarching statements of identity. Goals, strategies, policies, and operational guidelines are derivatives of these three statements. If the appointment of a board is the starting point in creating a group, the articulation of guiding principles is where the board's work begins. The interim board will initiate some of this work, but in all likelihood the overarching principles of the group will not fully coalesce until that early work is developed further by a permanent governing body. Even then, the principles are not static constructs. They need to be periodically revisited, modified as necessary, and reaffirmed, especially if the membership of the hospital affiliated group practice is growing rapidly.

Hospital- and system-owned practices are subject to a caveat that is not germane to independent, freestanding groups. In the context of institutional ownership, the group practice board's span of control is circumscribed. The group's mission, vision, and values will already have been shaped to some extent by the hospital's guiding principles. Also, the health system governing body may assign some of the authority traditionally vested in the boards of freestanding organizations to others in the system management hierarchy—for example, to the senior executive overseeing the group.

These nonnegotiable limitations and constraints may induce feelings of disempowerment in the members of an employed group's board. This sense of disempowerment results from a misunderstanding.

First, the presence of higher authority (the hospital or system) does not negate the importance of physician affirmation of guiding principles or of the physician board's advice. The importance of this advisory role cannot be overstated. The only way that corporate "owners" can expect to tap into the power of group practice culture is by taking the opinions of group members seriously and assimilating the group practice board's advice in setting health system policy and strategic direction.

Second, as group practices mature, most hospitals and health systems are eager to increase the authority delegated to the group practice board. Many forward-looking health systems even express intent to have the group practice board exercise a major role in leadership of the entire institution at some point. This arrangement is discussed at greater length in Chapter 13. Formal decision-making authority will be delegated gradually as the group practice board becomes more sophisticated and the group/hospital relationship more symbiotic.

Invariably, management first delegates clinical decisions to the group practice board because it is not in a position to make them itself. Examples include approving clinical protocols and pathways, setting the scope of practice guidelines, and addressing peer review matters. Authority over recruitment and retention decisions is the next power commonly delegated to the board. Many hospitals give their group practice boards veto power over recruits and defer to these boards in such matters as discipline and contract renewal.

DIFFERENCES BETWEEN THE GROUP PRACTICE BOARD AND THE MEDICAL STAFF

How do the prerogatives of the group practice board differ from those of the formal medical staff? When the medical staff has approved policies or procedures, group practice members are obliged to follow them (within the institutional boundaries of the hospital). Thus, with respect to inpatient practice, the policies and dictates of the group practice cannot contravene the medical staff bylaws or policies. They can, however, exceed or amplify requirements of medical staff membership for group practice members.

For instance, the group practice board can require that its members have a higher level of experience to receive a clinical credential than that required by the medical staff, but it can never create lesser standards. Additionally, because employed physician groups provide most of their care in nonacute settings—primarily physician offices— the group practice board will address a host of issues outside the jurisdiction of the medical staff, and the group's policies will hold sway in ambulatory settings where medical staff bylaws have no purview.

As the ranks of hospital-employed physicians grow in the nation's hospitals, it is important for these institutions to actively manage the "town-gown" conflicts that are inevitable. Practitioners in private practice are often fearful that the health system will favor the employed physicians. Such disgruntled physicians may seek control of medical staff positions as a way to exert power over the employed group. It is critical for the group practice to see that its membership stays active in the affairs of the hospital medical staff and does not cede this organization to the diminishing pool of private practitioners. In cases where the hospital affiliated group practice becomes a large portion of the medical staff, the group practice board and medical staff executive committee need to maintain a dialogue to avoid duplicating activities such as credentialing and peer review.

A PRIMER ON GOVERNANCE

The group practice board's sphere of authority involves two other roles—the group practice medical director and practice administrator. These individuals are responsible for organizing and managing all aspects of day-to-day practice.

There is a critical distinction between *governance* and *management*. Governance is about the big picture—creating a vision and setting goals. Management is about translating the big picture into a functional reality. There is an old tale about Noah and the ark that clarifies this difference:

> When Noah heard the weather forecast he ordered the building of an ark. (This is an act of governance.) Then Noah looked around and said, "Make sure the elephants don't see what the rabbits are up to!"(This is an act of management.)

The work of a governing board can be organized into four broad areas:

- Guidance
- Oversight
- Ambassadorship
- Self-regulation

Guidance

Guidance starts with an articulation of mission, vision, and values. While these statements seem generic, they have to be crafted carefully. Their language and tone need to reflect local concerns and commitments, and they need to be truthful and authentic. Board members need to feel enough sense of ownership that they are able to articulate these statements of principle with authority and personal conviction.

Guidance continues with the articulation of strategy and policy. Strategy is a synthesis of mission, vision, and values; business knowledge; and market intelligence. It asks, "What specific accomplishments (goals) will fulfill our mission, vision, and values, given the business realities and local market conditions in which we operate?" An employed group practice's strategies and goals should be tightly synchronized with the business plans of the hospital/system and consider the satisfaction and developmental needs of professionals in the group. The board may also frame tactics that will drive group success, but it will rely primarily on its medical director and practice administrator to devise and implement the tactical programs that turn strategic ideas into operational success.

The board is also the final decision maker about complex issues that define the character of the group or determine the group's direction. When contentious issues are brought to the board for final decision, or when issues are appealed to the board as a final arbiter of operational decisions, board members are not simply making isolated rulings but are translating overarching values into operational terms and setting policy precedents for the future.

Oversight

While the board delegates operational responsibility to its management team, it cannot delegate its responsibility for goal fulfillment. *Oversight* is the process by which the board ensures organizational performance without committing the cardinal sin of *micromanagement*—excessive involvement in operational detail. Oversight involves regularly and rigorously monitoring performance metrics associated with each of the organization's goals and each area subject to serious regulatory or legal constraints.

Adequate oversight cannot be exercised unless an organization's goals have been translated into metrics the board can gather and review. So that oversight can be efficient as well as effective, infrastructure needs to be built that will allow the necessary information to be gathered without undue difficulty. Increasingly, complex organizations are using two concepts to organize data flow to the board: the dashboard and the balanced scorecard.

Dashboards are telegraphic arrays of data that organize significant amounts of information into simple, clear displays. *Balanced scorecards*, developed by Harvard Business School professors Robert Kaplan and David Norton (1996), organize different types of data (financial data and quality data, for instance) in a way that shows their interrelationships.

The board's review of operational performance is not meant to be a passive process. It needs to be a rigorous exercise in which difficult questions are asked and action steps are framed to ensure success. Follow-up on those action steps and the results deriving from them complete the cycle of goal setting, oversight, new goal setting, and oversight, ad infinitum.

Ambassadorship

Board members' deliberations should be informed by a deep understanding of the issues—needs, concerns, and hopes—of group members. They also need to ensure that their formal decisions are disseminated, understood, and, as much as possible, appreciated by group members. For these reasons, outreach is critical and communication can never be overdone. Many successful boards make communication a regular agenda item at meetings to emphasize the importance of this activity.

While some board matters need to be kept confidential (e.g., disciplinary investigations or certain strategy discussions), the *process* by which the board considers these matters can be transparent. By using a transparent decision-making process, boards earn the trust of their constituents, even when the particulars of the case must remain private.

In addition to internal ambassadorship, the board has the important responsibility of representing the group to its many external publics—hospital or health system management, patients, payers, and the community. As a hospital's group practice grows larger and more sophisticated, elected leaders of the group practice have an important role to play by representing the group in health system strategy development. Board members may also participate in national groups such as the American Medical Group Association to showcase the group and learn from similar organizations around the country.

Self-Regulation

The fourth board function relates to nurturing and developing the board through education, self-assessment, attention to group process, selection and preparation of future board members, and, if necessary, development of policies that govern its work.

Periodic self-assessment allows the board to ask and thoughtfully explore critical questions such as the following:

- Are we helping the organization meet its goals?
- How might we improve the process we use to accomplish these goals?

- Can we improve the way we organize and review data, the quality of our discussions, and our ability to resolve conflict?
- Is the level of individual participation optimal?
- Are our committees effective?

Paul Dieckert, MD, previous chair of the Scott & White Board of Directors, perfectly captured this sense of the board's role in describing his own organization. See Exhibit 7.1.

LEGAL DUTIES OF BOARD MEMBERS

There are three legal duties associated with board membership:

- *The duty of care*: Board members must exercise thoughtful attention to their duties as described in the previous sections.
- *The duty of mission*: Board members must make decisions guided only by the goal of assisting the organization with mission fulfillment.

Exhibit 7.1 Governance at Scott & White

"The purpose of physician governance at Scott & White is to ensure that all major decisions by the leadership of Scott & White serve the well-being of our patients and advance the practice of compassionate, scientific medicine. Physician governance at Scott & White enables recruitment and retention of highly qualified physicians, nurses, and professional managers, whose dedicated teamwork is translated into excellence in patient care. The commitment of our physicians to self-governance is a key aspect of our identity, and a cornerstone of our success."

J. Paul Dieckert, MD
Chair, Board of Directors 2005–2008
Scott & White Clinic

- *The duty of loyalty*: Board members must act for the highest good of the organization by acknowledging potential conflicts of interest and maintaining confidentiality.

FUNDAMENTAL PRINCIPLES OF GOOD GOVERNANCE

- *The board speaks with one voice.* While disagreement in the boardroom is healthy and important, the board's determinations guide the organization, so it needs to provide one set of directions. Public expression of dissenting opinion and minority reports are not acceptable. Differences of opinion must be negotiated and resolved within the boardroom. Resolution commonly takes the form of compromise, synthetic opinions, or contingency plans.
- *The board considers constituent concerns but is not representational.* Inevitably, each board member will have specialized knowledge (e.g., a surgeon understands how the group's ambulatory surgery center functions). Just as inevitably, each board member will have a vested interest in a particular organizational outcome (e.g., preference for one model of reimbursement allocation among specialists and primary care physicians over another). While sharing unique knowledge and articulating the special interests of constituencies in the group are appropriate, board members' decisions should be based solely on the collective good, as defined by the mission of their organization.

BOARD COMPOSITION AND COMMITTEE STRUCTURE

There is a general consensus that to facilitate robust discussion, boards should comprise no fewer than 7 members and no more than

12. Boards with fewer than 7 members aren't diverse enough to have credibility, and boards of more than 12 members are generally too large to be effective.

Most boards' committee structure mirrors their areas of primary focus. The initial committees described in Chapter 6 may be supplemented, as the group evolves, with a separate finance committee, a benefit options committee, or a professional affairs committee (to deal with professional development, discipline, and peer support). Hospital affiliated group practices rarely need to appoint an executive committee, unless political realities have forced the creation of a board that is too large to be effective. A regular or ad hoc nominating committee can help ensure that the right group members are elected to the board. Some committees can be designed to include members who are not part of the board. Such design provides an opportunity to mentor potential future board members and increase the transparency of the board's activity.

The board needs to clearly communicate its expectations to each committee and define the limits of the committees' authority. Committees need to advance the projects assigned to them but should not co-opt the prerogatives of the board. While committees can (and should) make recommendations, only the board has the authority to make decisions for the organization. Thus, all committees have a balancing act to perform—they need to do enough work to provide real value, but they need to be careful not to pre-empt the board's jurisdiction.

THE GROUP PRACTICE GOVERNANCE LEARNING PROCESS

Physicians tend to have little experience in organizational leadership and a poor appreciation of the role a board plays. Physicians who grew up (professionally) in the traditional medical staff structure often had to work with cumbersome, unfocused committees that attended to procedural details rather than overarching issues of identity, policy, and strategy.

Already biased toward a focus on details (because the practice of medicine requires such a focus), group practice board members are at risk of developing the wrong habits as a result of their early experiences in organizational life. Governance education and steady coaching of new group practice boards are essential to ensuring that attention is directed toward governance matters—overarching concerns and big-picture issues.

An ad hoc or standing nominating committee can help ensure that those elected to the board are prepared for their new roles. First, this committee can establish nominating criteria to de-politicize the election process and help group members make more informed and thoughtful decisions. Second, the nominating committee can identify potential future board members and direct the group's medical director to provide these individuals with a steady stream of opportunities to develop leadership skills. Finally, the nominating committee should create a rigorous and formal orientation for new board members to speed up learning as much as possible.

THE UNIQUE ROLE OF THE CHAIR

While the board chair does not have an operational role (operations being the province of the group practice administrative team and medical director), the chair is the "face" of the group—internally and externally—and has a critical role in articulating the group's values, vision, and operating principles. He or she needs to be visible, articulate, politic, and relatively "unflappable."

Speaking for the board, the board chair inputs the perspective of the group practice to senior hospital/health system administration, guides the work of the medical director, leads board meetings, and conducts public forums. The board chair may also serve as an ex-officio member of the health system board. Behind the scenes, a lot of work goes into these simple tasks. Board meeting agendas need to be set, the data stream to the board needs to be shaped, presentations to the board need to be directed, committees need to be guided in their work, and board members need to be coached. Coaching and providing feedback to fellow members are not easy tasks for new board chairs; such mentoring runs counter to medical groups' strong culture of egalitarianism. If the chair cannot guide his or her colleagues toward making their best contribution, however, they often remain without guidance.

All of these duties may require a board chair to step well beyond his or her previous level of organizational sophistication. In such cases, the chair needs to arrange for the support—coaching, development, and education—he or she needs.

Occasionally, the board chair also serves as the medical director. This practice is unwise for two reasons. First, profound confusion about the difference between governance and management will inevitably result. Second, for the reasons articulated in Chapter 6, the medical director should be hired through an interview process, not selected via a voting process.

COMPENSATION FOR THE WORK OF GOVERNANCE

Given the importance of the board, and that most group practice compensation schemes focus on rewarding productivity, the work of governance should be recognized by compensating board members. There is some debate as to whether stipends should be based on the job or on what a physician might earn in the office. (The latter model would vary according to specialty.) Most groups set a uniform stipend for all members.

Chairs, particularly those of large groups, usually receive larger stipends. Their compensation also may increase during the intensive start-up phase of smaller groups, when they often work half-time or more on organizational matters.

CONCLUSION

The governing body is the heart and soul of a hospital affiliated group practice. Administrators expect the board to contribute to the system, and group members trust that it will advocate for physicians appropriately, communicate effectively, and guide wisely. Excellent governance can go a long way toward ensuring group success. Conversely, a weak, misguided, or confused board is a major risk factor and portends significant difficulties in group performance over the long run.

CHAPTER 8

Group Practice Leadership

THE TOPIC OF PHYSICIAN LEADERSHIP surfaces repeatedly in discussions about health system effectiveness. Why? What is so magical about physician leadership, as opposed to other types of leadership? Is it that different from the general topic of leadership, which has been the subject of hundreds of thousands of business books?

WHY PHYSICIAN LEADERSHIP?

From their matriculation into medical school until the culmination of their postgraduate education, physicians are trained to embrace the responsibility of making life and death decisions. No matter what changes about clinical practice, what specialty a physician chooses, or what preoccupations interfere with a physician's professional life, this fundamental responsibility defines what being a doctor means.

As Bujak (2008) and others have described, physicians are inclined, as a result of the subtle process of acculturation into medicine, to be suspicious of collective decisions, to focus on the needs of individual patients rather than the collective needs of populations, and to assume that traditional business algorithms are unlikely to be relevant to their clinical work.

These beliefs and behaviors set the stage for physicians to be skeptical at best, disdainful at worst, of nonphysician leadership. This attitude is not unique to the medical profession; other groups that undergo intense professional training, particularly concerning matters of life and death (e.g., the military or the police), assume a similar posture.

For these reasons, physicians are unlikely to accept the authority of leaders unless they, too, are physicians. This reality makes physician leadership essential for healthcare organizations. But how do we ensure that accepted leaders are also competent leaders?

THE RISE OF THE PHYSICIAN EXECUTIVE

Academic institutions, which are organized around deans, departmental chairs, and practice plan directors, have perhaps the longest tradition of physician leadership. Outside of academia and physician-owned facilities (including traditional freestanding large group practices), there was little professional physician leadership of large health institutions until the 1980s. In most hospitals, the elected officers of the medical staff provided what leadership they could without formal training or clear authority other than that assigned by the hospital and medical staff bylaws.

Through the 1980s, the growing complexity of the medical enterprise increasingly strained hospital–physician relationships (see Chapter 1), and hospitals turned to a new leadership role—vice president for medical affairs (VPMA)—for help. The VPMA was often a respected member of the medical staff, someone close to retirement and politically neutral, whom the hospital could rely on to conduct "shuttle diplomacy" when conflicts emerged. The VPMA initially had little formal training in management and leadership, and little formal accountability within the executive team.

Over the 1980s and 90s, the role of the VPMA became increasingly complex, and educational opportunities for physician leaders became more readily available. For decades, the American College of Physician Executives has led groundbreaking efforts in this regard.

As a result, physician leadership has changed dramatically over the last 30 years. Today's physician executives are likely to be tasked with real operational responsibilities and to have been prepared for those tasks via a series of supervised developmental experiences, formal educational programs, and advanced degrees.

Many systems have replaced the VPMA with a chief medical officer (CMO) or created a CMO position to oversee (among other duties) VPMAs at multiple hospitals. Often hospitals create additional medical directorships to address specific physician groups or clinical service areas. These physicians may be employed under an exclusive contract with the hospital, those involved in a specific hospital service line (e.g., orthopedics or neurosciences), or the doctors who work in a particular section of the hospital, such as the emergency department or intensive care unit. The following sections will show that the use of such medical directors is ubiquitous in large, successful independent group practices, where they are often assigned by specialty or geographic region.

LEADERSHIP COMPETENCIES OF THE PHYSICIAN EXECUTIVE

Many of the skills required of physician executives are generic, common to any leadership position in any business. These skills include the ability to work on a team, communicate effectively, understand business planning and business finance, manage change, deliver performance reviews, empower others, and manage accountability.

In addition to these fundamental skills, physician leaders need to be knowledgeable about areas specific to the medical enterprise. These areas include quality and safety, clinical workflow design, healthcare financing, the proper use of clinical guidelines, health information technology, public health, and physician compensation. Physician leaders also need to be skilled at motivating and mobilizing their colleagues, who often feel beleaguered and alienated from the same hospitals seeking to partner with them. A sample leadership curriculum is outlined in Exhibit 8.1.

Beyond didactic training, physician leaders invariably need to be supervised and mentored, but these activities are often neglected. Senior hospital and system leaders are reluctant to supervise and mentor physician executives and often defer to them unconsciously because these tasks would be inappropriate in *clinical* situations. In management situations, however, supervision and mentoring are critical. The senior health system executive responsible for the group practice should not shy away from this task and should employ external coaches as needed to supplement hospital-based resources. Coursework, no matter how useful, is a poor substitute for supervision and mentoring. As the hospital affiliated group grows, its success will in part depend on how well its medical director supervises and mentors the practice's growing, decentralized leadership team.

Exhibit 8.1 Selected Topics for a Physician Leadership Curriculum

- The nature of leadership
- Governance versus management
- Managing change in organizations
- Running effective meetings
- Organizational cohesion: group dynamics; legal and human resources issues
- Quality, safety, and risk management
- Rapid cycle process improvement
- Problem solving and crisis management
- Communication and conflict resolution
- An introduction to health economics
- Physician compensation
- Marketing and branding
- Health and society: major issues in public health
- Health reform: key issues and ideas

GROUP-FOCUSED VERSUS HOSPITAL-FOCUSED PHYSICIAN LEADERSHIP

Physician leadership in the employed group practice and in the "parent" hospital or health system operates in distinct but overlapping domains. The hospital VPMA has a portfolio of duties that focus on the inpatient facility as well as the ambulatory programs and satellites the hospital controls. The VPMA also supports the medical executive committee of the hospital medical staff, whose responsibility and authority are limited to inpatient practice and hospital-controlled outpatient venues.

The leadership of the group practice will need to work closely with the VPMA and medical staff leaders wherever its members are involved in traditional hospital activities. However, much of the work conducted by the employed group will take place in ambulatory settings, outside the purview of the medical staff and the traditional VPMA. The group's leaders will have to deal with issues like ambulatory practice structure and physician compensation models that have no correlate inside the hospital. For these reasons, the skill mix and focus of group practice leaders will be different than that of their inpatient colleagues.

SELECTING AND DEVELOPING THE GROUP PRACTICE MEDICAL DIRECTOR

In addition to the president or chair elected by the group practice board to convene its members and organize its work, the board and responsible system executive recruit a medical director to oversee the group practice's operations.

In general, this position should not be filled on a part-time basis by the hospital VPMA or health system CMO. Neither of these executives is likely to have adequate time or focus to fill this role. Group practices tend to recruit medical directors from within. Internal appointment is less threatening to physicians because they are already familiar with the nominee's management style, and health system administrators prefer not to deal with an outsider who doesn't know the system. The group/system may further rationalize internal recruitment by claiming that too much change can be problematic and that the nominee can acquire any missing skills over time.

This political approach slows the pace of change and does not serve groups well. The task of building a strong, successful employed group is best approached boldly and enthusiastically. This contention does not imply that the medical director *must* be an outsider, but rather that this person must demonstrate his or her competence as a leader, commitment to the task of group formation, and willingness to develop the skills required of the role.

The search process should not begin with a review of incumbent physicians who might fit the role. Appropriate candidates cannot be identified until a description of the job has been articulated and criteria have been set. The board and senior executive responsible for the group should partner in this search and reach consensus before proceeding with any decisions.

Groups that identify multiple strong internal candidates may choose to forgo a national search for purposes of expediency. Even in such cases, though, a national search can be educational and can reassure the group that the incumbent it selected was the best candidate.

The new medical director's learning curve will depend on his or her strengths and weaknesses. In most cases, internal recruits will need exposure to other systems to broaden their experience. They will need to be coached, encouraged, and supported to take on a different role with familiar clinical and administrative colleagues. They may need to supplement their repertoire of existing skills so they are able to deploy the full set of competencies required of the medical director. External recruits will need to be mentored closely as they catch up on years or even decades of learning about the culture in which they have landed.

Newly appointed medical directors—whether internal or external candidates—also need to commit time and energy to building the relationships they will need to leverage their skills and experience.

Physicians who acquired leadership experience from working in a medical staff structure are likely to rely on personal relationships and political levers for influence. These physicians will need help developing skills and comfort with managerial approaches of leading, including goal development, empowerment, and assignment of accountability.[1]

THE MEDICAL DIRECTOR'S RESPONSIBILITIES AND REPORTING RELATIONSHIPS

The medical director's job is to ensure that the group's physicians translate into practice the mission, vision, values, and strategies articulated by the board and hospital. The medical director reports to the group practice board and often has a "dotted line" of accountability to the hospital/health system executive responsible for the group's performance. (See Exhibit 8.2 for a sample organization chart.) This individual is also a major conduit of communication between the group practice and leaders throughout the hospital, medical staff, and health system.

Invariably, the medical director will need to work closely with the nonphysician expert or team of experts that drives the group's practice management activities. In some groups, these administrators report to the medical director. More often, they report to the system senior executive who oversees the group practice. Regardless of the reporting structure, the relationships between the medical director and his or her administrative counterparts need to be open, mutually respectful, and collaborative. As expressed in the quote by the CEO of Ochsner Medical Center in Exhibit 8.3, such cooperation between physician and management leaders creates a cultural foundation of mutual accountability.

There is much debate as to whether physician executives should maintain a dual role of clinician and administrator. Those in favor

Exhibit 8.2 A Typical Organizational Chart for a Large Employed Medical Group

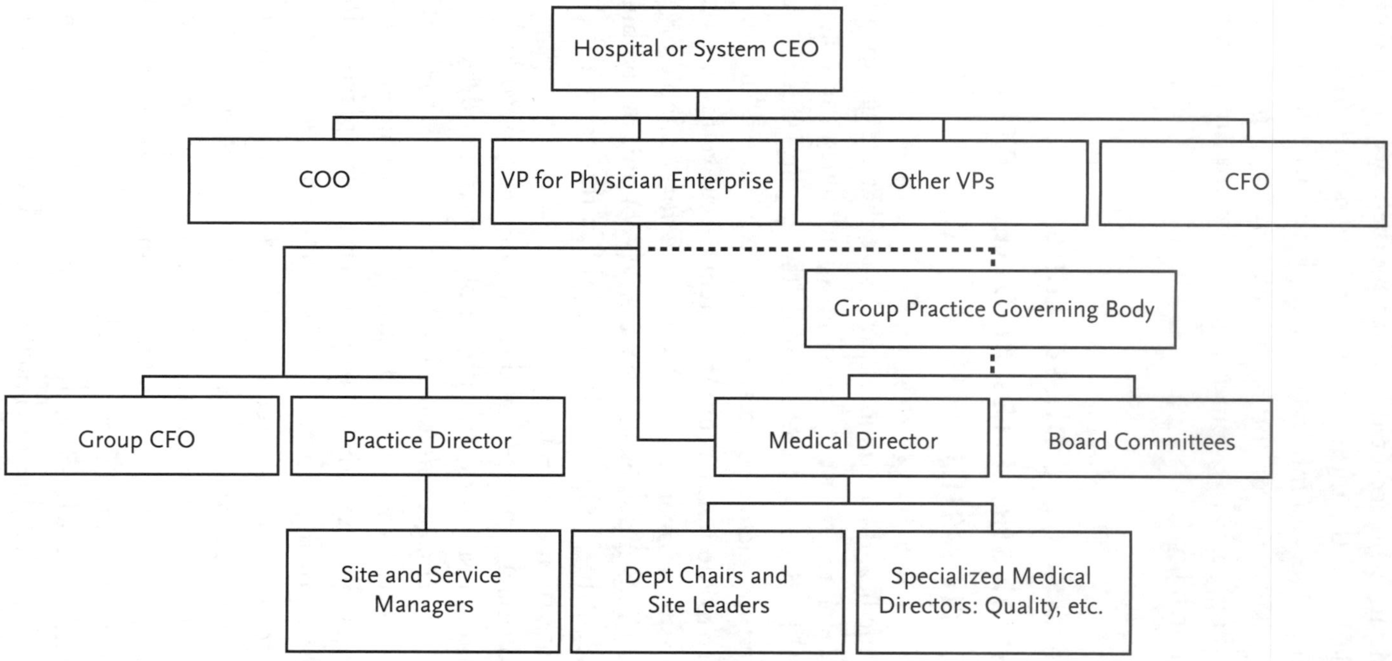

Hospital or System CEO

COO

VP for Physician Enterprise

Other VPs

CFO

Group Practice Governing Body

Group CFO

Practice Director

Medical Director

Board Committees

Site and Service Managers

Dept Chairs and Site Leaders

Specialized Medical Directors: Quality, etc.

Exhibit 8.3 Accountability and Culture at Ochsner

"In our group practice, we work to foster a culture where the members of the group think like owners.... This is very evident in our strategic planning process. Every year, each department chair and their administrative counterpart do a rolling three-year strategic plan....

"The physician leader and administrative counterpart jointly present their plan to the medical director and myself. This fosters a culture whereby the physician leader and administrative leader are accountable to each other, to the organization, and to the other members of the group....

"This planning process with the physician leaders in our group means we are planning with the leaders of the group, not for them."

Mike Hulefeld, CEO
Ochsner Medical Center

assert that a physician executive should continue to practice to maintain credibility and a sense of identity. Further, the size of an employed group in its early stages may not warrant a full-time medical director. Medical directors comfortable in their roles and able to relate to the concerns of practicing colleagues, however, can usually maintain credibility without continuing clinical work. If they no longer practice, though, they should be aware that their physician colleagues may consider them "out of touch." They should be prepared to demonstrate their appreciation of practice issues and deal graciously but authoritatively with those who challenge their credibility.

Personnel Management

While every medical director's job description is different, this role is always charged with two major areas of responsibility: personnel and performance management. The medical director is involved in recruiting, inducting physicians into the group, credentialing, assigning doctors to sites in the group's service area, providing performance evaluation and feedback, taking disciplinary action, and promoting professional development (which includes identifying and nurturing those capable of becoming future leaders). He or she also must have good problem-solving skills to be able to deal with unpredictable yet inevitable issues, including malpractice, illness, and interpersonal conflict.

In large groups, the medical director may assign these tasks to other leaders or create committees for these purposes. Examples include a recruitment committee that interviews candidates, an orientation committee that mentors new recruits, a professional affairs committee that investigates issues of behavioral or clinical competence, a credentialing committee, and a wellness committee that supports physicians struggling with health issues or substance abuse. While committees can be useful, the scope of their authority (advisory versus decisional) and the manner in which they are appointed (chartered by the board or empanelled by the medical director) must be clear.

Recruitment

The group practice should have a plan for growth that is tightly coordinated with the hospital or health system's medical staff development plan. The medical director implements this plan not only through recruitment activities (e.g., reviewing applications and interviewing) but also through induction and mentoring (to orient and acculturate new physicians). When there are problems with a new recruit, the medical director is usually responsible for identifying the problem(s) and designing appropriate remediation. If the problems persist despite corrective efforts, the medical director initiates the process for termination without undue delay. An expeditious resolution is in the best interest of both the practice and the new recruit.

Performance Management

Every group practice needs to have a process for regular review of its practitioners' performance, including quality, productivity, and conduct. Regular review also provides an opportunity for discussion between the medical director and each physician. While this ritual is common in most work environments, physicians are not accustomed to it. The medical director (and performance review committee, if applicable) needs to be mindful of this unfamiliarity and approach this task with some delicacy.

The medical director must initiate corrective action when mentoring and regular feedback fail to foster adequate professional performance and citizenship. The employment contract should identify events that can trigger such action, and consequences, including termination of employment, should be detailed in the group's policies. The relationships between corrective actions taken by the group practice and those imposed by the medical staff are discussed in Chapter 12.

After ensuring, in the words of Jim Collins (2001, 13), that the group has "the right people on the bus," the medical director must keep the bus driving in the right direction. The following dimensions of performance are especially important in a multispecialty group practice:

- Productivity
- Utilization
- Conformance with quality and patient safety benchmarks
- Liability reduction
- Patient access and service
- Process improvement

Productivity

The medical director should regularly monitor productivity on an individual, departmental, and work area basis, solve problems as necessary to create structures and processes that support expected performance, and help the group's physicians establish a work rhythm that is productive and personally gratifying. The medical director must also address circumstances in which high individual productivity may be undermining quality. For example, under a compensation model that emphasizes payment for throughput, a physician might inadvertently sacrifice patient safety or patient satisfaction by treating patients too quickly.

Utilization Management

Utilization management has always been a concern for groups that treat a large managed care population. With value-based purchasing, it becomes a concern for every provider organization. When interventions must be made to address poor utilization performance, a group practice's physician leaders should explore systemic reasons for the problem and/or confront the practitioner in question if individual practice issues are the problem.

If the group is the sole provider of professional services under an at-risk contract, the medical director will need to build a structure to oversee care delivery and utilization for that contract. In some large groups, such tasks are delegated to a "managed care medical director," who reports to the group medical director.

Quality and Safety

Quality and safety processes in ambulatory practice are not nearly as developed and accepted as would be ideal. American medicine could (and should) show much better results with regard to quality and safety (Institute of Medicine 2000, 2001). As payment is increasingly linked to quality and safety outcomes through various pay-for-performance metrics, the economic viability of health systems and their employed or affiliated group practice(s) will be tied to achievements in this area. The group medical director should be responsible for working with the board and appropriate committees to set quality goals, orchestrate improvement efforts designed to meet those goals, monitor performance, and provide group and individual feedback on how performance compares to benchmarks.

Risk Management and Incident Review

The medical director typically plays a key role in risk management and incident review. Until hospital-employed groups reach considerable size, hospital-based departments may provide administrative support for these functions. The medical director and senior executive responsible for the group must ensure that these departments devote adequate time to the needs of the group, develop the skills necessary to work effectively in ambulatory settings, and fully involve the group medical director as a partner. In many cases, hospitals and health systems that self-insure will transfer the malpractice liability policies of employed doctors from private insurers to the hospital plan. Large groups often have a dedicated risk management staff that reports to the medical director and the system CEO or general counsel.

Access and Service

High levels of access and service are key drivers of group success. If patients cannot see their providers when they have concerns, or feel poorly treated when they do have appointments, they will seek alternative care. As financial responsibility shifts to patients through higher copayments and deductibles, institutional vulnerability to patients' choices increases. The medical director is often charged with designing systems of care that optimize the patient's experience and helping colleagues appreciate the importance of commitment to patient service by teaching them necessary skills.

Process Improvement

Demands for service, quality, and efficiency all require that we design more effective ways of practicing medicine. The cohesion and culture of group practices present unique opportunities to reinvent approaches to care delivery to achieve superior results. The medical director can be influential in catalyzing creative projects in care design and helping to spread innovations in one area throughout the organization.

AS THE GROUP GROWS: LEADERSHIP DEVELOPMENT AND INFRASTRUCTURE

Large group practices require tiers of leadership (Lister 1998). One medical director will not be able to do all that is necessary as the group grows beyond 80 physicians. There are two ways of approaching the development of an extended physician leadership group. The first is to appoint medical directors to areas of particular concern, such as quality, managed care, and service improvement. These positions, usually part time, report to the group practice medical director.

More commonly, duties are assigned to department chairs, who carry out managerial duties along specialty or service lines. Groups that have practice sites in numerous locations may also appoint local practice directors. Local leaders can address issues unique to their practice site or clinical specialty more expeditiously. All these positions should report to the group practice medical director.

As duties and responsibilities are disbursed among a larger, decentralized leadership team, role definition and scope of authority must be kept clear. Two principles need to be reconciled:

1 Local solutions need to be crafted through dialogue with those affected.
2 Solutions should be uniform across the group practice *when uniformity yields value.*

This arrangement requires that a balance be struck. Local leaders should be empowered to make decisions but also held accountable for doing their part in meeting the group's overarching goals. The medical director needs to be available to these leaders as a resource but learn not to accept "upstream delegation." Instead, local and departmental leaders should be coached and equipped with the skills they need to address problems in their areas on their own. Just as supervision and mentoring are critical to the medical director's development, the medical director must embrace the role of supervisor and mentor for all the group's leaders.

As a group grows, role clarity is not the only issue. The priorities of the medical director start to shift. The selection, development, and supervision of subordinate leaders become higher priorities. Over time, departmental and geographical physician leaders must become increasingly effective at working with their own administrative partners to solve local problems and initiate local improvements. Working as a coordinated leadership entity, these physician–administrator teams share best practices and address interdepartmental challenges collaboratively. As these teams grow in their abilities, less hands-on management will be required of the medical director. Instead, his or her role will involve overseeing innovation efforts, coordinating the work of other leaders, ensuring consistency where necessary, and leading enterprise-wide initiatives.

CONCLUSION

Successful development of a sophisticated leadership infrastructure for a large or decentralized group hinges on identifying and preparing a substantial cadre of leaders. This task should begin in the early stages of a group practice's formation. Current and future leaders should be prepared through a common curriculum. This education should also provide developing leaders with opportunities to interact with colleagues at off-site meetings. External exposure prevents the group's knowledge base and assumptions from becoming parochial, familiarizes the group with the best practices of other institutions, and acquaints group leaders with helpful contacts from across the country.

NOTE

1. See Lister, E. D., and A. Czerwinski, "Leadership in Action: Improving the Decision-Making Processes of Medical Group Practices," *Group Practice Journal* (51): 6, June 2002.

CHAPTER 9

Culture: The Bonds That Hold the Group Together

IN ADDITION TO GOVERNANCE and leadership, culture is an indispensible, unifying ingredient of healthy groups. Culture is not a fixed property of medical groups or any other organization. It can emerge and morph spontaneously, or it can be cultivated carefully. When forming a new group practice, leaders must be mindful and deliberate about the process of culture building.

WHAT IS CULTURE?

Group members need to share values and commitments, which translate into behavioral expectations and performance. Without attention to the development of desired culture, hundreds of physicians, trained to be autonomous, will not unify automatically. Shared commitments are more important to group cohesion than economic interdependence. Without this glue there is no group, only the pretense of one.

The next time you are in a hospital waiting room, observe what's going on around you. Do staff members pick up trash from the floor? Do they greet patients as they come in? Do they make eye contact? Does anyone notice the lost, confused patient? Each action (or inaction) is a manifestation of culture. Culture drives an organization to be patient-centric or physician-centric, to be safety conscious, to strive for excellence, to be respectful of everyone in its community, to be team-oriented, or to demonstrate a number of other behaviors.

While not inclusive, the following list highlights key dimensions of group culture. Each parameter can be defined in terms of both norms (expectations) and behavior.

- *Collegiality*: How do physicians refer to each other (e.g., by reference to specialty, or as colleagues or partners)? Do they help each other, communicate promptly, make decisions collaboratively, and confront difficulties directly? What happens if one physician asks another for an urgent consultation at 4:45 p.m. on a Friday? Is a gracious response expected? Is it the norm? Does the group have formal guidelines that define expectations for civil and collegial behavior?
- *Patient-centeredness*: Is the rhythm of the organization geared around patients' needs versus technological efficiency or physician convenience? Can a patient see multiple physicians in the same office in one visit? Are patients viewed as partners in their care?
- *Proactivity*: Is the group committed to identifying opportunities for improvement and experimenting with change before problems fester? Does the group frequently demonstrate behaviors supporting this commitment?
- *Empowerment*: Do the group's top leaders encourage local leaders to invent solutions to local problems (as opposed to referring everything up the chain of command)?
- *Accountability*: Are physicians held accountable for their performance and behavior? Does the group have a regular review process? Can it cite situations in which problematic performance was dealt with promptly and effectively? Is accountability maintained through a respectful, collegial process or a "shame and blame" approach?
- *Innovation*: Is energy regularly invested into creating new and

better processes? Are there examples of individuals or teams that have done so and been recognized or rewarded?

- *Balance (centralization/decentralization)*: Are local problems solved locally? Are policies consistent across the organization? Are strategic decisions made in the best interest of the *entire* group, and after a comprehensive quest for input?

CULTURAL BUILDING BLOCKS

Culture is created and sustained through action. In established societies, most of this action is carried out unconsciously. For example, parents are not required by law to read morality tales to their children. They do so because it is common practice and "the right thing to do." Group practices are not naturally occurring social formations, however, so the values that create and sustain group culture need to be planned and implemented.

In the previous section we described seven dimensions of group culture. The discussion that follows describes eight *tactics* for building group practice culture and shows how each is germane to propagation of that culture.

Recruitment

Physicians selected for the group should have an understanding of—and affinity for—collective practice. This attribute is unrelated to technical competency and clinical knowledge. Questions that explore attitudes as well as aptitudes should inform the recruitment process. References need to be queried about the candidate's ability to collaborate, willingness to engage in collective problem solving, willingness to compromise, and communication skills. The best groups disqualify candidates who are not interested in collaboration and interdependence, even when these physicians have a strong background of clinical excellence.

Induction

Induction is the process by which new members are brought into the group and expectations are presented and clarified. Induction is typically achieved through a thoughtful orientation program and communication of written group practice expectations. The latter is sometimes encompassed in a formal group practice covenant (discussed later) that articulates what group members expect from one another.

Mentoring and Modeling

The mentoring process helps new physicians become acclimated to the group. Physicians should be mentored for the first 6 to 12 months of their employment. Regular meetings with an established physician who embraces the group's values can be informal—over coffee or dinner—but cannot be neglected. These meetings, casual observation and feedback, and role modeling illustrate and reinforce the expectations presented upon formal induction into the group.

Performance Review and Feedback

Without regular feedback, most people have difficulty recognizing problems and changing behaviors appropriately. Regular, formal review of individual performance data promotes and sustains a group culture of self-improvement and excellence. As part of this process, each physician, working with an appropriate group practice leader, should explore the two-sided question of how he or she can make a greater contribution to the group and, conversely, how the group can improve the physician's professional satisfaction.

In the best of groups, physicians have enough commitment to group norms that peers can deliver feedback spontaneously (e.g., "Sam, are you OK today? You seem to be off your game."), instead of "going up the ladder."

Variable Compensation

Group practice compensation schemes are primarily designed to reflect market rates and reward individual productivity. Most long-standing groups also reserve funds to reward performance in other areas, such as citizenship, service, and quality. If a group does not have a system that rewards physicians financially for performance in these areas, its compensation scheme, by focusing solely on productivity, discredits those values.

Office Design

The organization of physical space can support or undermine efforts to build cultural attributes, such as collaboration. Physicians should be colocated in a space that structurally emphasizes the interdisciplinary nature of the group.

Process Design

The design of group processes, like that of physical space, can support or undermine group values. Does the practice have a common system that allows physicians from different departments and office sites to approach their work in a consistent manner? Shared information systems, central scheduling, and common referral and communication systems are essential to group unity. The use of similar performance metrics, feedback systems, and problem-solving templates also promotes a consistent approach to work across the enterprise.

Process Improvement

Successful groups pay significant attention to where and how they can improve. Some focus on adopting quality improvement technologies from other industries (e.g., the Lean approach of Toyota, or Six Sigma management); others concentrate on eliminating the historical approach to process improvement of blaming and inducing fear, seen so often in American hospitals. Whatever approach they use, process improvement is part of these groups' culture. Their members share a commitment to improvement and—just as important—a willingness to embrace change.

CREATING CULTURE—THE EARLY STAGES OF GROUP FORMATION

By the time a hospital decides to pursue development of an integrated group practice, it usually already employs a number of physicians. These individuals and/or practices were often acquired as a defensive or opportunistic effort to prevent their defection from the community, prevent their acquisition by a competitor, secure a vital service line, or retain an important referral base. The hospital likely put little thought into whether they would fit in an integrated multispecialty group practice.

These employed physicians should be actively engaged in conversations about the intent to create a different structure and culture. Ideally, they will be excited about this prospect and willing to guide the initiative to ensure that the group develops the cultural attributes listed in the previous sections. As discussed in Chapter 5, the work of group formation is complex and will require that incumbent physicians be shown examples of high-functioning groups and then be both inspired and coached to create a similar environment.

Some of the hospital's employed physicians will have little interest in, or little aptitude for, transitioning to a more centralized organization committed to coordinated patient care and an interdependent business model. Through redoubled effort, an attempt must be made to engage these physicians in the group development process. If this attempt fails, frank discussions may be necessary about moving forward with group formation without these physicians. They will have the option of returning to self-employment or continuing in an employed relationship with the hospital, outside of the group practice.

The transition from "employed physician" to "member of an employed group" is fundamentally a shift toward engagement. Employed physicians are simply asked to deliver clinical service. Members of a group practice are asked to participate in creating a culture that will be sustained by their involvement in a wide variety of activities beyond clinical practice, and to practice in a way that reflects the group's cultural values.

How will an increased level of physician engagement be achieved in this second wave of practitioner employment, and how will group formation drive that process? To this end, two levels of motivation need to be tapped.

The first is self-interest. As discussed in Part I of this book, physicians are seeking employment positions with hospitals partly to attain secure and attractive compensation. One lesson hospitals learned from the first wave of physician employment is that compensation should be tied to productivity. In contemporary employment situations, compensation should additionally be tied to the added value physicians bring to the health system. If organizational goals are met and the system's bottom line improves, these gains should be reflected in the compensation paid to physicians. This arrangement incents doctors to engage actively and meaningfully in the group's initiatives. (Compensation arrangements are discussed in more detail in Chapter 10.)

The second motivation is physicians' sense of professionalism and idealism. Regulatory difficulties, reimbursement frustrations, and practice complexities can turn the joy of practice into a distant memory. Pressure to be productive results in hurried appointments, and subspecialization results in clinical encounters focused on organ systems rather than more holistic interactions with patients.

As discussed in Chapter 5, hospitals and systems that create strong physician groups aim to transform healthcare. The power to excite and revitalize physicians, seen in the best of groups, stems from this audacious goal. When physicians are given the opportunity to drive change across the system, the gains in quality, efficiency, and patient service can be remarkable.

To accomplish such change, physicians must be constantly reminded of the vision of the integrated enterprise and their role in fulfilling it. They should be given examples of successes achieved in the best-performing integrated group practices around the country and challenged to generate examples of their own. A onetime presentation during the recruitment phase will not inspire momentous change. Physicians should be given repeated opportunities to contribute toward this vision, and their achievements to this end should be regularly recognized and celebrated. This approach sets in motion a self-perpetuating cycle of engagement.

SUSTAINING CULTURE IN AN EXISTING GROUP

Recruitment into an Existing Group

Once an institution commits to growing the group practice, recruitment criteria should be quickly established. In some markets, physicians who understand the opportunity posed by hospital employment may rush to climb on board. However, as already noted, some physicians are not good matches for an integrated group practice. Discipline is required to turn away a physician or medical practice that wants to join but would be inappropriate. With the board aiming to protect the culture of the group, and the senior administrator responsible for the group arguing for the economic advantages of adding another doctor, such decisions are often marked by tension.

A consistent recruitment process and clear guidelines, agreed upon in advance by the board and senior administrator, help to manage the balance between protecting culture and fostering growth. These guidelines should address the following questions:

- Will this physician be a good team player?
- Does this physician have leadership potential?
- Can this physician maintain good working relationships?
- Does he or she have a good track record with regard to patient satisfaction?
- Can this physician take direction from physician leadership, or must he or she always be in control?
- Does he or she have good communication skills?
- Is this doctor computer literate or willing to learn to use an electronic medical record?
- Do other physicians on staff have confidence in this doctor's clinical skills, or do they tend to refer elsewhere?
- Are there incidents of unprofessional conduct in this doctor's past?
- Does the physician buy into the vision of the integrated delivery system?
- Is the physician comfortable with the group's compensation formula?

To increase the chance of finding good fits, the group would be wise to recruit from the ranks of physicians already accustomed to a group practice setting. Such individuals may have practiced in the military or a public health setting, come from a staff model HMO, or have experience as a member of another group practice.

Although the recruitment process has historically been driven from the administrative side, the senior administrator should partner with the medical director when recruiting for the group and enlist the support of a physician recruitment committee. The recruitment committee should make recommendations to the group's board and the senior practice administrator, who are responsible for formal contracting.

This committee is important for several reasons. First, it brings rank-and-file physicians into the process, furthering their sense of engagement and self-determination. Second, committee involvement demonstrates a commitment to group norms and gives multiple physicians an opportunity to evaluate a candidate's potential to fit within the group. Third, the committee can demonstrate to applicants that membership in the group practice is a positive experience. Finally, committee involvement prevents applicants who have been turned down from circumventing the administrator in charge of recruitment and appealing directly to their physician colleagues. In addition to compromising the group's criteria for inclusion, such behavior can invoke disunity between the group's doctors and the administrator who supports the practice.

MISSION, VISION, VALUES, AND A GUIDING COVENANT

The group's governing body is responsible for drafting a mission, vision, and statement of values for the practice. These statements should be crafted in a way that overpowers the cynicism physicians tend to express when presented with lofty statements of principle. While these statements must be compatible with those of the parent system, they also can capture some essence of the group's beliefs and perspectives. By articulating and revisiting its mission, vision, and values, the group reinforces its commitment to these principles.

Harry Levinson, one of the pioneers of organizational psychology in the United States, developed the concept of "the psychological contract" (see Chapter 3) in a way particularly useful to this discussion (Diamond 2003). This concept refers to the unwritten, often unconscious behavioral expectations between employer and employee in any workplace. His work suggests that much can be gained by making these unspoken agreements explicit. Many organizations that ascribe a high value to teamwork and integration apply Levinson's wisdom by articulating a mutual commitment between the group practice and its physician members, called a *covenant*. Some of the most successful group practices create a covenant as a natural extension of their mission, vision, and values. An example of a covenant is provided in Exhibit 9.1.

Exhibit 9.1 Sample Covenant

Riverside Medical Group* Physician Covenant

We will focus on patients as our first responsibility.
- Practice evidence-based medicine
- Encourage patient involvement in care and treatment decisions
- Achieve and maintain optimal patient access
- Insist on seamless service

We will collaborate on care delivery.
- Include all members of the interdisciplinary team in treatment decisions
- Treat all team members with respect
- Demonstrate the highest levels of ethical and professional conduct
- Behave in a manner consistent with team goals
- Participate in and support teaching

We will listen and communicate constructively.
- Communicate clinical information in a clear, timely manner
- Request and/or provide information on resources needed to deliver care
- Provide and accept feedback, and hold each other accountable for the quality of care we deliver

We will take ownership.
- Implement RHS- and RMG-accepted clinical standards of care
- Participate in and support group decisions
- Understand the economic impact of our decisions on patients' access to care
- Recognize our fiduciary responsibility to support RMG and RHS
- Encourage community involvement

We will change.
- Embrace innovation and continuous improvement
- Participate in organizational change
- Commit to lifelong learning

*Riverside Medical Group (RMG) is part of the Riverside Health System (RHS) in Newport News, VA. Used with permission.

Leadership is responsible for modeling the commitments the group has set forth, promulgating the message, and reversing any group drift from these values and commitments.

DEALING WITH CONFLICTS AND BEHAVIORAL DIFFICULTIES

Conflict in groups is inevitable. Social scientists have noted that every culture has a consistent way of dealing with conflict that is an amalgam of historical practices and values. Two types of conflict boards commonly encounter are disagreements about 1) direction and 2) the need to discipline a member of the group. In choosing how to approach these matters, the board has an opportunity not just to reflect accrued culture but also to shape it.

Whether disagreements about direction are strategic (should we enter a new market?) or tactical (should we rearrange patient flow in our office?), they are bound to occur. Physicians typically advance their opinions with a lot of passion but often do not have sufficient knowledge or perspective to justify their positions. Group leaders should embrace a decision-making process that can be modeled and consistently applied. The following steps can be used as a template in designing this process:

1. Articulate the problem or opportunity.
2. Identify those accountable and responsible for resolution.
3. Request input and ideas.
4. Agree on the criteria for decision making.
5. Gather data and seek expert opinion as necessary.
6. Synthesize the best options.
7. Weigh multiple options against preestablished criteria (select a group of neutral individuals for this step, if necessary), and decide on a policy or action.
8. Present the proposed plan of action for feedback and approval

(where necessary) by the committee, board, or responsible executive.

9. Communicate the decision and the rationale by which it was reached to all concerned.

Problem-solving skills (soliciting input; creating synthetic solutions) can be formally taught and regularly practiced by using such a template. It ensures that the loudest voice will not trump the rest and that the issue will not close until it is carefully reviewed.

Disciplinary problems are also inevitable when individuals interact in a large group over an extended period. Complaints from patients, hospital personnel, peers, or people outside the workplace can expose problems. As described earlier, a covenant that clearly articulates group expectations provides a standard against which behavior can be compared and judged as problematic or benign. In addition to a covenant, most group practices, as most medical staffs, benefit from having a code of conduct that explicitly describes unacceptable behaviors and corresponding consequences.

When confronted with allegations of behavioral difficulty, the group must balance its members' due process rights and its commitment to act in their best interest with the need to protect the norms and values of the group as a whole. Action must be fair, confidential, and expeditious. While the principle of confidentiality usually precludes explaining to group members the details of the rationale for a disciplinary decision, reviewing the fairness of the process with them is appropriate.

Groups should have policies that describe a consistent process for the investigation of allegations of behavioral difficulty and steps for selecting an appropriate intervention. Members' rights to appeal those decisions must also be clear. Policies should also specify a continuum of potential consequences (e.g., ranging from admonition to dismissal). Leaders should follow up on every intervention to ensure that the disciplined party has amended his or her behavior.

Inexperienced group practice leaders tend to avoid conflict and tolerate inappropriate behavior because "it wasn't that bad." Such justification and inaction are demoralizing for the group and all of its external publics (including support staff) and communicate a lack of concern for the well-being of its members. In contrast, rigorous but fairly enforced standards tend to build morale.

Leaders would be wise to keep two additional guidelines for the disciplinary process in mind. First, the group should not rely on the disciplinary mechanisms of the hospital medical staff because (1) problematic behavior may not have occurred in a venue within the medical staff's purview and/or (2) the medical staff's standards may be different from those of the group. An ability to handle such issues internally is a hallmark of an effective group practice. Second, because groups are usually subject to the personnel policies of their hospital employers, group processes should be designed within the framework of the hospital's human resources department and legal counsel.

In disciplinary matters, predictability and dependability engender trust and loyalty, whereas inconsistency based on politics undermines group members' confidence, sense of safety, and willingness to commit to the practice.

THE CULTURE/QUALITY/SAFETY LINK

U.S. hospitals are paying a great deal of attention to quality and safety and the cultural commitments that foster these attributes. By embracing the need for improved care delivery and greater attention to quality and safety, the group practice can not only lead critical hospital or system initiatives but also demonstrate its commitment to patient-centered care and professional values.

The National Patient Safety Foundation and others have drawn attention to the role culture plays in advancing quality and safety initiatives, emphasizing the need to evolve from a "culture of blame" to a "culture of fairness."[1] This transformation encourages employees to identify mistakes and potential problems, sharing them so that systematic changes can be implemented to prevent their recurrence. To help organizations in these efforts, the Agency for Healthcare

Research and Quality has developed a survey to assess safety culture in a hospital setting.[2]

A proactive focus on quality and safety interrupts the cycle of external criticism and mandated change that can be demoralizing to physicians. The nation's leading group practices focus relentlessly on leading the pursuit of quality, beginning with attention to supporting quality and safety efforts via the assertion of appropriate cultural expectations. Emanating from that commitment is a willingness to measure and document the results of quality and safety efforts, the steady pursuit of innovation, and impatience with "business as usual."

CELEBRATION AND RENEWAL

To sustain connectivity between group members, rituals must be established that bring them together to collaborate and celebrate. While maintaining a proud and successful group culture through such rituals is enormously rewarding, it is also hard work. A lot of planning is required to convene all members of a group. The increasing value younger physicians place on family and/or personal time after work hours makes this feat even more challenging.

Nevertheless, convening is critical. Colleagues scattered across an extensive geographic marketplace cannot get to know each other personally if they do not gather together regularly. Transportation, hotel, and child care expenses for physicians who do not live near the meeting location need to be seen as essential business costs, and leaders need to encourage attendance.

Festivities need not be exorbitant. A simple party can be held to celebrate the group's values and accomplishments and honor members who have contributed to its success. Spouses should be invited to the festivities so they, too, feel included in the culture. Spouse involvement reinforces members' connection to the group and may increase their desire to remain with the group long term.

The leadership infrastructure described in Chapter 8 is essential to maintaining a sense of cohesion in large groups. When leaders convene regularly, know each other well, and collaborate in problem solving and cultural development, they will have less difficulty surmounting the barriers posed by size and distance. For example, a physician can approach the leader he or she knows best and ask, "I need to refer a family to a pediatrician in our other practice site who works well with nervous parents, but I don't know anybody there. Can you consult your counterpart there and find that physician?"

CONCLUSION

The importance of culture in transforming an organization and sustaining the changes over time cannot be overemphasized. An old business school aphorism says, "Culture eats strategy for breakfast every day." Without culture, the group may have little to show for its best-laid plans and achievements.

NOTES

1. See the National Patient Safety Foundation's mission and vision statements at www.npsf.org/au.

2. See www.ahrq.gov/qual/patientsafetyculture.

PART III

CHAPTER 10

Delivering on the Promise of Integrated Care: Infrastructure, Business Operations, Finance, and Compensation

THE ADVANTAGES OF PHYSICIAN EMPLOYMENT and evolution to a group practice model must be carefully leveraged and sustained by a sophisticated infrastructure. This lesson hit home during the first wave of physician employment in the 1980s, when financial losses caused the employment model to collapse. The power of the group needs to be used to generate financial rewards for both the host institution and the group.

CREATING AN OVERALL STRATEGY FOR THE GROUP

Most small office practices accommodate change reactively and do not create forward-looking strategic plans. Hospital affiliated group practices should anticipate the need for change and plan for it proactively. Practice leadership should create a thoughtful strategic plan early in the stages of group formation and update it on an ongoing basis. This plan needs to be constructed with the overall strategic agenda of the health system clearly in mind and designed to support that agenda. Such foresight keeps members mindful of the group's ambitions and intentions for the future and can be used to benchmark progress toward fulfilling those aims.

The strategy also will need to take into account the history leading up to group formation. No two hospital affiliated groups are the same, and no two institutions follow the same path to group formation. Many hospitals build around a nucleus of primary care providers, while others are propelled by employed specialists. Some start with a cadre of independently employed physicians. Others begin by assimilating an established community group practice. In addition to considering current conditions, leaders should "begin with the end in mind"—in other words, give significant thought to what kind of group will support the hospital or system strategy five to ten years downstream.

The following list includes examples of questions that group decision makers can use to guide the formation of a strategic plan:

- What is the right mix of specialists for the group?
- What should be the geographic "footprint" of the group? (Where should offices be located, and how many are needed?)
- What is the desired rate of growth for the group?
- Should the group practice develop "programs of excellence" and seek program certification where available?
- Should the group practice establish multispecialty office sites that promote "one-stop shopping" for patients?
- Should the group practice implement the "medical home" as a delivery model, as advocated by many health policy organizations?
- As the group grows in size and complexity, should it organize its infrastructure around specialty departments or multidisciplinary service lines?
- Should established practices be allowed to retain their names or some "subgroup identity" when incorporated into the hospital affiliated practice?
- How competitive should the group practice be with private practitioners in the community?

- What level of leadership should the group practice provide for hospital service lines?

RATIONALIZING THE GEOGRAPHICAL PLACEMENT OF PHYSICIANS AND THE STAFFING OF PHYSICIAN OFFICES

Physicians recruited from private and small group practices into hospital employment are often assured implicitly or explicitly that they will be able to maintain their status quo. Such guarantees are the kiss of death to group practice formation because they imply a commitment to physician autonomy and self-interest over collective success. Assuring recruits that participation in a hospital-owned group is a path to a rewarding and stable professional life is different from guaranteeing that particular details will remain unchanged.

Two areas in which tensions often arise are retention of office space (particularly if it is physician owned) and retention of office staff. The comfort of accustomed space and familiar, accommodating staff is not easily surrendered.

Operational efficiency is required to sustain a practice, and clusters of ambulatory offices work better in this respect than smaller, randomly scattered offices. Beyond capturing efficiencies, bringing physicians together so that they can work in close proximity to each other has a powerful impact on the group's cohesion and its ability to serve its patients, as the quote in Exhibit 10.1 attests. The location of these larger ambulatory sites should not be left to chance but strategically placed to reflect the competitive landscape, population density, and patient travel patterns.

What can the group offer physicians to attenuate the loss of comfort involved in leaving their professional homes? Allowing some personalization and customization of office suites can significantly increase a doctor's willingness to relocate. When designing new office space, every physician who will practice there should be given an opportunity to provide input. Physicians new to the group should feel from the start that they are participants in shaping their future.

The ideal group practice site is not just a collection of offices under a superstructure but an integration of practice areas colocated with strategic support services. Physicians of like specialty should be clustered in areas that allow staff and resources to be shared.

Every effort should be made to create multispecialty office buildings that provide one-stop shopping for patients. In addition to large collections of physician offices, these facilities can house diagnostic testing sites (e.g., radiology and laboratory services), pharmacies, and social service providers. The advantages such facilities offer, such as easy access to the expertise of colleagues in close proximity and quick diagnostic testing, can help distract new members of the employed group practice from becoming nostalgic about the loss of their previous offices. They are also likely to find they have more satisfied patients. See Exhibit 10.1 on the Palo Alto Experience.

Staff issues are likely to be more of a challenge than physical office relocation. Employees, particularly longstanding employees, will be anxious about a change of practice ownership and are likely to have little experience juggling loyalty to "their doctor" with allegiance to a larger institution. In many cases, staff members of private practices were previously employed by the hospital or health system and left in favor of work in a small, more personal, and less bureaucratic office setting. Ground rules should be established before these staff members are absorbed into the employee pool of the hospital-owned group practice. The most basic of these ground rules is acceptance of direct accountability to a practice manager or practice management team charged with overseeing the entire ambulatory network of the group practice. A willingness to work within—and become a part of—such a structure should be a precondition to continued employment.

A second critical ground rule is commitment to work beyond the confines of a single office. Practices are more cost-effective and efficient when their staff members are "interchangeable" and can cover others' responsibilities in cases of absence (e.g., vacations, unexpected

Exhibit 10.1 Colocation: The Palo Alto Foundation Medical Group Experience

"The relationships that develop by working shoulder-to-shoulder caring for patients help physicians to make tough administrative decisions together. Collaborating on patient care dramatically increases our ability to collaborate on the more difficult organizational issues.

"It is hard to overstate the importance of aligning incentives for all stakeholders in a group, and of breaking down the walls (literally) that foster silos based on geography or specialty.

"This leads to a culture of jointly diagnosing, and developing treatment plans for patients, as well as organizational challenges. Fully developed, this supports the creation of a shared group vision."

(P. F. DeChant, MD, president, Palomares Division, Palo Alto Medical Foundation, personal communication)

---

illness) or other needs, both anticipated and emergent. This commitment requires staff members to rethink their roles as supporting not just one physician but the entire group.

The final ground rule is a willingness to embrace change. Staff must be amenable to letting go of their traditional work methods. One of the great strengths of large group environments is the ability to take best practices proven in one area and spread them throughout the organization.

The organization's needs and expectations for staff must be clearly communicated to physicians entering employment so they can coach incumbent office help in the skills and attitudes essential to future success. When practice managers evaluate staff members at the time of office conversion and thereafter, they need to solicit input from the practice's physicians and apprise them of staff performance evaluations. Such inclusion increases the likelihood that physicians will feel they are part of the management structure of the group they have joined. It also wins physician buy-in to the expectations the group has for staff and maximizes the chances that staff will successfully convert to employment in the new group setting.

BRANDING, MARKETING, AND SERVICE

Strategy meets the public through the group's branding and marketing activities. Branding unifies the group through physical means (e.g., colocation of practices, signage, logos, decorating schemes, scheduling processes, billing practice, uniforms). Marketing communicates to the public that this group practice has integrated solutions to all family health needs. Both functions announce that the health system, hospital, and group practice have interlaced a dizzying and confusing array of treatment options to offer patients a seamless, coordinated, user-friendly experience.

This message is sustainable, of course, only if the level of service provided "delivers" on the promise of integration. Staff members at every level need to reference the wholeness of the group and take responsibility for ensuring patients a seamless experience. The statement "After admission, you are going to be taken care of *by my partners* on the hospitalist team…" is much more powerful than "I'll be referring you to the hospitalists…."

One challenge that hospitals encounter when they market their employed groups is independent practitioners' jealousy and, sometimes, anger. These physicians, who may be loyal to the hospital and important to the hospital's economic success, are inclined to perceive the hospital's efforts as providing an unfair competitive advantage to the employed portion of the medical staff. To defuse this tension, hospitals would be prudent also to market the practices of independent providers who are engaged in and aligned with the hospital's mission and vision. Instead of emphasizing integration, however, marketing for independent practices should focus on provider skill and availability. Outreach to non–group members is discussed further in Chapter 13.

INFORMATION TECHNOLOGY

An integrated electronic health record (EHR) shared by all group members and staff is a practice's "central nervous system." Implementation of such a system should be one of the highest priorities of hospitals and systems committed to realizing the full potential of employed physicians. Many of the efficiencies referenced in the sections and chapter that follow depend on a system's ability to share and extract information effortlessly.

Hospitals need to move quickly to an integrated solution that includes clinical, practice management, and revenue cycle modules. One challenge in this process is finding software that can communicate across inpatient and outpatient systems, or at least support bridges and interfaces that maximize data sharing.

Hospitals should expect to invest significant capital in creating a comprehensive IT platform for the group. Physicians need to be involved in planning so they can help shape the system. Physicians will be more willing to use a system if they have influenced its design. Willing or not, however, all members of the employed group should be required to use electronic record keeping, without exception. This requirement should be made clear early in the recruitment process.

Difficulties may arise when existing community practices folded into the hospital affiliated group already use a different EHR. Physicians who have invested time to learn one system will be resistant to throwing out a perfectly good EHR to accommodate the product chosen by the hospital. While maintaining multiple EHR systems in one group might seem to be the path of least resistance, it increases the expense of technical support and reduces the possibilities of seamless interoperability. Here again, clear expectations about migration to the group practice EHR needs to be established from the outset with new recruits.

PRACTICE MANAGEMENT: APPROPRIATE CENTRALIZATION AND STANDARDIZATION OF OFFICE PRACTICE

Hospitals may be loath to create another bureaucracy to manage the activities of a new group practice. They may be inclined to reduce costs and complexity by using hospital managers already responsible for various outpatient operations. However, successful hospital affiliated group practices need to have key administrators who are expert in office practice management and who understand how to run large sites, as well as multisite practices. Site- and specialty-specific staff must understand their reporting relationship to these administrators. A seasoned practice director with responsibilities across the group ensures uniform human resource policies, efficient and consistent deployment of staff, and common administrative processes across sites of service.

Some of the greatest gains in efficiency and clinical effectiveness are made through office standardization. Yet when presented with the idea of building and standardizing the group practice according to a set of imposed practices, physicians may resist and chafe at what they consider intrusions into the way their offices are run. The practice director must be empowered by the practice board to achieve this goal.

There are several keys to engaging physicians and staff in office standardization:

1. Clarify expectations when physicians enter the practice. When physicians are recruited with the promise that nothing will change, they respond to any requests for practice efficiency as though they have been deceived.
2. Involve physicians and their preexisting staff in designing office practices and capturing best practices, and have them work with their peers to reach consensus on optimal approaches.

3. Create incentives. Reward creative ideas and initiative. Calculate the cost of delivering service—by encounter or by relative value units (RVUs)—in each office setting. (RVUs are a measure of the work effort expended by the physician in caring for a patient.) Consideration should be given to allocating any discretionary funds available under the compensation formula to providers who can minimize the cost of delivering service while maintaining throughput, service, and quality. To the degree it is under physician control, cost per RVU of service delivered should be relevant when calculating physician compensation.

4. To foster buy-in from staff and physicians, be explicit about the rationale for standardizing processes.

5. Differentiate clearly between issues that require standardized *processes* and issues that require standardized *outcomes*. Requiring all practice sites to deliver high levels of patient care is reasonable; requiring every receptionist to greet a patient with the same words is not. When allowed to customize some office processes, physicians and office staff are more likely to tolerate standardization of others.

6. Clearly communicate that staff will be required to "float" (i.e., provide coverage across practice sites) and that some degree of standardization will be required for this reason. Staff members should be rewarded when they translate time spent in different offices into ideas for practice-wide process improvement.

SET APPROPRIATE EXPECTATIONS BY BEGINNING WITH A REASONABLE ECONOMIC MODEL

There is nothing more demoralizing to employed physicians, or the practice directors working with those physicians, than to be told repeatedly that they are losing money when the hospital's economic model makes profitability impossible. Are losses on employed physicians inevitable? If so, why? The answer depends on the way hospital executives perceive the economics of hospital-employed or affiliated physicians. The following are important points to consider when shaping this perspective:

1. Expecting to recapture the costs of buying a practice, let alone with some return on investment (ROI), is unrealistic. This lesson became clear in the 1980s. Today physician practices are purchased for the value of receivables and hard assets only. Paying for goodwill on the basis of past earnings is unwise; doing so sets dangerous precedents, and economic return is highly unlikely. If incentives such as practice purchase arrangements and signing bonuses are needed to entice physicians into employment, these outlays should be seen as investments in infrastructure (i.e., costs of doing business) that are not expected to be recouped later through the physicians' revenue stream.

2. Physician practices are rarely profitable without ancillary income, which is why every freestanding group practice does all it can to bring ancillaries in-house, whether that ancillary is a simple lab in a two-person family practice group or a nuclear camera in a cardiologist's office.

3. Hospitals have two choices: They can direct all ancillary income to traditional hospital departments or allocate certain ancillary revenue streams to the group. Most hospital-owned practices direct all testing to inpatient facilities, and the health system allocates facility fees exclusively to the hospital department rather than to the group. Ultimately, the choice is irrelevant, as long as the operating budget constructed for the group is realistic in the context of this decision. The performance of the group needs to be measured in terms of realistic expectations, given the overall economic benefit to the health system, and not simply in terms of positive or negative cash flow. For example, in many instances, billing/collecting for ancillaries under the hospital's billing number results in

increased reimbursement based on negotiated fee schedules and contracts. Doing so reduces income attributed to the group but maximizes it for the health system.

4. Regardless of the economic model for ancillary revenue, there is a compelling argument for placing dedicated diagnostic equipment in the physical location of the group practice, rather than having the group use hospital-based equipment. Ambulatory patients often experience substandard customer service when they are directed to inpatient facilities, as schedules inevitably yield to the needs of patients with more severe or emergent conditions. Also, the development of the group practice brand is often boosted by dedicated ancillary services when they can be delivered in a personable and patient-centered way. These considerations may be less relevant for small hospital-owned groups but become compelling when hospital-owned groups grow to 70 physicians or more, particularly as practices become colocated.

5. Strategic investments need to be differentiated from operating investments. Clustering the group's physicians makes for more efficient practice administration. However, marketplace dominance is often advanced by a more widely dispersed placement of ambulatory sites of service. If the hospital and its group decide to sacrifice efficiency for strategic purposes, it cannot expect to recoup the strategic investment in short order. Again, expectations and budgets need to be set accordingly.

6. Operational issues are different. A practice that requests more examining rooms should be able to justify the expenditure through a straightforward business plan, with a simple ROI analysis. The same distinction between strategic and operational investments should apply to decisions about major purchases, such as the purchase of an EHR.

7. Payer mix issues must be considered. Stand-alone ambulatory practices are profitable to the extent that they (a) reduce their panel of Medicare and Medicaid patients (because the rate of payment for these patients usually lags that of private payers)

and (b) don't provide care for the uninsured. Hospitals, however, may depend on Medicare patients and, in some instances, have negotiated profitable rates for certain Medicaid services. *System* success often requires optimum utilization of inpatient facilities, which in turn requires that the hospital's group welcome elderly and disabled (Medicare and Medicaid) patients.

8. Despite the economic consequences, most health systems extend themselves to the underinsured and uninsured as a way of meeting the requirements of their service mission. Often they ask physician members of their employed group practice to assume clinical management of these patients. Asking the group to carry a disproportionate share of this responsibility can offer economic relief to independent physicians and play a significant role in winning their support.

9. Revenue expectations need to be articulated in a way that reflects these policies, and members of the group practice need to feel rewarded, rather than penalized, for helping their hospital and community by being open to all classes of payers. This calculus translates to a need for the hospital-owned group practice to work in a "payer-blind" way, accepting all or most insurances. In doing so, two critical budgetary considerations must be made. First, income expectations for the group need to be set in a way that realistically reflects payer mix. Second, providing incentives to practitioners to treat patients with better rates of reimbursement is counterproductive. For this reason, most group practices use a compensation formula that focuses on RVU production rather than on billings or receipts.

THE ART OF BUDGETING

The considerations discussed in the previous section suggest that realistic and transparent budgeting is critical to group morale and evaluation of practice success. The creation of an appropriate accountability loop holds both practice administrators and physicians accountable for what they can control but does not expect them to deliver results that are not achievable under the group's fiscal model.

Budgets need to be built around expected revenue (estimated on the basis of the anticipated payer mix) in the context of appropriate productivity standards and anticipated practice costs. The group budget should involve productivity targets, cost targets, and compensation that can flex with marketplace changes or alterations to system strategy. Physician compensation needs to track regional benchmarks for similar levels of productivity by specialty and be designed to reward desired behavior.

Expectations also need to be set for downstream revenue, including incremental volumes of diagnostic tests, medical admissions, and surgeries. To fully evaluate the group's economic impact, the hospital or system needs to develop the ability to quantify its contribution to inpatient and ancillary revenue. Group efforts that save the hospital expenses (e.g., rationalizing equipment purchases or streamlining an approach to care delivery in a service line) also should be recognized as group contributions.

PREPARING FOR NEW TRENDS IN REIMBURSEMENT

Various iterations of pay for performance (P4P) have been in place for years now and will become ever more exacting. P4P methodologies will unquestionably continue to expand from the inpatient arena to ambulatory care settings, with different payers focusing on different aspects of prevention, chronic disease management, and early intervention. More complex P4P strategies stress the need to coordinate care across ambulatory and inpatient settings, and some reward caregivers for preventing the use of emergency facilities. In addition, three other "value-based" methodologies—bundled payments, gain-sharing, and use of the medical home to provide coordinated care—are receiving considerable attention from the Centers for Medicare &

Medicaid Services (CMS) and the Medicare Payment Advisory Commission (MedPAC) as this book goes to print.[1]

These demands and related payment strategies create enormous opportunities for hospital-based group practices to fully deliver on the promise of integrated care. For example, the concept of bundled payments is a reimbursement scheme in which a single payment is made for an array of clinical services delivered by multiple providers, for a defined episode of care, for a patient diagnosed with a specific condition. Such "global case reimbursement" would cover the services provided by the hospital, inpatient and outpatient physicians, pharmacies, imaging centers, and laboratories. The approach involves a degree of risk sharing among these entities and emphasizes the role integration has in the emerging reimbursement climate. Exhibit 10.2 outlines the advantages available through integration.

PHYSICIAN COMPENSATION

In freestanding multispecialty groups, the unanswerable question of what is "fair" makes compensation a complex and charged issue. How should ancillary revenue be divided? How should compensation be allocated among primary care physicians and specialists? When should market considerations trump strict productivity formulae? How should administrative and citizenship contributions be measured and rewarded? These questions elicit only a few of the factors that make compensation decisions difficult. Controversy may be mitigated if the health system buoys group member compensation by attributing a portion of health system revenues to the efforts of the group practice. Hospital-owned group practice leaders may also insulate themselves from these tensions by relegating difficult compensation decisions to the hospital's administrative team.

Inevitably, though, as group practices mature, and because physicians tend to like to be in control, practice leaders will want to have more sway in compensation decisions. While the services of a compensation consultant are usually necessary to sort out the details

Exhibit 10.2 Optimizing Reimbursement under Pay for Performance and Bundling Payment Mechanisms

Factor Favoring Optimal Performance	Relevance	More Likely with a Group Practice?	Notes
A culture of teamwork and problem sharing	Providers compose a team and share a commitment to common care delivery goals.	Yes	See Chapter 9.
Case management bridging ambulatory and acute care	Decisions fully consider clinical options.	Yes	Traditionally, hospital case managers have no influence on ambulatory care.
The ability to create unitary charges for complex and multi-provider encounters	A unitary payment scheme anticipates need for billing reform, transparency, and comparability across provider organizations.	Yes	Group and inpatient billing, contracting, and revenue cycles would have to be integrated.
A common EHR across sites of service	A common EHR is critical to optimal information transfer.	Yes	
Full teamwork among hospitalists and outpatient providers	Teamwork minimizes the impact of transfers and hand-offs.	Yes	An emphasis on shared responsibility underlines the importance of having hospitalists in the group practice.

(Continued on following page)

(Continued from previous page)

Factor Favoring Optimal Performance	Relevance	More Likely with a Group Practice?	Notes
Medical leadership infrastructure that encompasses the continuum of care	This structure is conducive to problem solving, conflict resolution, and coaching.	Yes	See Chapter 8.
The ability to create a relatively simple compensation strategy for those involved	Adoption of such a strategy makes alignment of incentives more likely	Yes	While "fairness" of compensation is a complex issue, group practices have an ethos that embraces and rewards teamwork and integration of care (see Chapter 9).

of compensation plans for large multispecialty groups, we have found several principles to be universally relevant:

1. Physicians won't trust a compensation plan unless it is transparent and consistent. Salaries need not be public, but the process by which they are set needs to be manifest.
2. Barring strategic reasons to the contrary, base productivity calculations should be determined by RVUs rather than by billings or collections for reasons itemized earlier.
3. The majority (70 to 90 percent) of established physicians' compensation should be based on productivity. The compensation rate relative to a given level of productivity needs to be set on the basis of the market rates paid for a given specialty in a given region.

4. Compensation for new physicians beginning a practice, physicians with significant administrative roles, and physicians assigned a role of strategic importance (stationed at a new site of service, for instance) should not follow this formula because such assignments compromise a physician's ability to be productive.

5. Compensation for the remaining 10 to 30 percent should be tied to citizenship, service, and quality on the basis of algorithms created by group practice leaders. The collective success of the group in meeting its budget targets may also influence this discretionary dimension of compensation.

6. Some groups focus on the cost of care as well as physician productivity or revenue generation. They divide shared overhead equally or according to a set formula that might, for instance, pass a greater burden to more highly compensated proceduralists. They then create a category of overhead separate from this shared overhead, usually called "direct overhead," which encompasses individually chosen benefits and extra staff support and is allocated directly to the providers who elect these conveniences. For example, a physician who prefers to have two assistants instead of one would be directly responsible for this additional overhead. This bifurcated approach to overhead allocation maximizes members' individual control but becomes increasingly unwieldy as groups grow. If this approach is used, the calculations involved should be made as simple as possible.

7. In general, all sources of income should be considered parts of total compensation.

8. Opportunities to moonlight outside of the employed group and earn supplemental income should be carefully circumscribed and subject to administrative permission, if allowed at all.

9. Part-time administrative physicians should receive a stipend for administrative duties but otherwise participate in the same compensation system as everyone else.

10. Clear responsibilities for practice building should be set for new physicians whose income is protected by salary guarantees. They should also be assigned other important tasks (e.g., outreach, protocol development, chart review) to perform during open slots in their schedules.
11. Physicians whose ability to be productive is compromised "for the good of the group" (e.g., with board approval, a third urologist is added in anticipation of growing patient volume, resulting in less work for the two incumbents) need some protection from the short-term consequences of such revision.

A thorough description of physician compensation plans is beyond the scope of this book. We encourage readers to consult the numerous publications produced on this subject by such organizations as Medical Group Management Association (MGMA) and Healthcare Financial Management Association.[2]

THE BASICS OF CODING AND CHARGE CAPTURE

Healthcare tabloids consistently report stories of physicians and health systems brought up on charges of fraudulent coding. These stories have a chilling effect on practicing physicians and all too often lead them to "under-code," driven by the rationale that it is better to be safe than sorry. There is little margin for error in either direction, however. "Over-coding"—that is, exaggerating the complexity of the delivered service—is unethical and fraught with legal consequences; under-coding threatens economic stability. Groups have struggled to find ways to incent physicians to code properly. Tying physician compensation to productivity rewards avoidance of under-coding but does nothing to caution against over-coding.

The only way to address this problem is to educate physicians on an ongoing basis and perform regular coding audits. In many organizations, the latter tactic has shown to be effective. In a coding audit, each physician's data are displayed to the group. Under- and over-coding are quantified, and the physicians see how accurately they are coding in comparison to their peers. This methodology harnesses physicians' competitive instincts and shows practice leaders where they need to focus remedial attention. As an incentive, prizes can be awarded for accuracy. Because charts must be reviewed frequently for this methodology to work, it may be criticized as excessively costly. In rebuttal, we can say with certainty that the potential cost of unmonitored practices would be far higher than the cost of ongoing audit practices.

RISK MANAGEMENT AND LIABILITY INSURANCE

When care is integrated and delivered by providers who share a common culture, leadership structure, and EHR, fewer adverse clinical events are likely to occur and the rate of malpractice claims is likely to decrease.

To realize such outcomes, the group practice needs to build a risk management function that is different from that of the hospital—that is, one that emphasizes ambulatory care and the ambulatory/inpatient interface. Although separate, the group's ambulatory-based risk management function and the hospital's inpatient-based risk management function should be tightly coordinated.

Further, the group should establish information systems and clinical protocols to ensure appropriate screening of incidents, recall of patients where necessary, and follow-up. Lessons learned need to be communicated throughout the group and hard-wired into practice. Risk management experiences need to drive quality and safety initiatives, which in turn should translate into practice expectations for every department and site of service. As discussed in chapters 8 and 9, leadership and culture in a group practice create value by making expectations for quality and safety explicit and embedding these expectations in the fabric of the group.

Many hospitals choose to include their employed group practices in a "captive" insurance strategy that reduces malpractice premiums. These savings benefit the hospital and can be shared with physicians via their compensation pool. The experience of Scott & White, one of the nation's largest group practice–based health systems, gives testimony to what a group can do by aggressively managing risk. See Exhibit 10.3.

TEACHING AND IMPLEMENTING RAPID CYCLE IMPROVEMENT

Most small physician office practices are case studies in inefficiency. Everyone generally works hard, but the constituent steps in patient registration, care delivery, and back office function have

---

Exhibit 10.3 Scott & White Health System Achieves Dramatic Results in Reducing the Cost of Insuring Clinical Risk

"A group practice provides dramatic advantages from a risk management perspective.

"Based on how the group functions, the overall risk profile of the group can be substantially reduced. We have seen the cost of medical malpractice fall steadily over the years, even in the face of rapidly expanding clinical volume."

(L. L. Havens, RN, JD, director of risk management, associate general counsel, Scott & White Memorial Hospital, personal communication)

---

rarely been studied or improved systematically. Standardization of these fundamental building blocks of practice efficiency is important to group practice success. Physicians and their staffs need to be involved in discussions about efficiency goals. As stated previously, distinction needs to be made between practices that need to be standardized (e.g., sterilization techniques) versus practices that need to achieve standardized goals (e.g., screening for depression), regardless of how the goal is met. Site visits to exemplary offices and staff rotation can accelerate the rate of improvement.

Practice leadership needs to learn and import to each office the skills involved in rapid cycle improvement (RCI). There are many "trademarked" RCI approaches. At the time of publication of this book, Six Sigma and Toyota's Lean production system are two popular techniques. Commitment to some form of ongoing process improvement is a critical success factor for any group. Physicians and staff across the entire clinical enterprise need to learn the necessary concepts and skills (ideally in small groups that cut across care delivery sites) and embrace process improvement as an intrinsic part of medical practice. In many situations, operating efficiency and clinical outcomes can be improved simultaneously.

CONCLUSION

Hospital administrators tend to underestimate the complexity of managing the business affairs of a large group practice. Physicians also tend to be unprepared for these challenges. As a consequence, many community-based multispecialty group practices have foundered. To guard against undesirable outcomes, experienced group practice managers from successful large groups should be hired when establishing a new hospital affiliated group practice. Close collaboration between hospital executives, physician leaders, and experienced group practice managers, coupled with steady, informed execution, is necessary to realize a substantial return on the time and resources invested in group development.

NOTES

1. For more information on bundled payments and value-based pricing, access the MedPAC website at www.medpac.gov.

2. A good example is the publication titled *Physician Compensation Plans: State-of-the-Art Strategies* by Johnson and Keegan, published by MGMA in 2006.

CHAPTER 11

Delivering on the Promise of Integrated Care: Clinical Operations

CLINICIANS AND CLINICAL SERVICES can be organized to exploit the latent advantages of group structure. The level of rigor prescribed in this chapter cannot be achieved without strong governance, leadership, and culture. Credentialing and appropriate privileging of practitioners, a robust peer review process, initiatives to implement strong clinical protocols, and attention to the utilization of resources are all required to sustain strong clinical operations.

CREDENTIALING, PRIVILEGES, AND INTERFACE WITH TRADITIONAL MEDICAL STAFF FUNCTIONS

In the traditional hospital setting, the credentialing and privileging process is a fundamental duty of the organized medical staff and a cornerstone of any organization with high-quality practitioners. In recent years, external regulators, accreditation agencies, and an increase in negligence lawsuits have motivated hospitals to apply more rigor to credentialing activities. Today, medical staffs with strong credentialing programs appoint members and grant them privileges on the basis of evidence rather than assumptions or pedigree.

As hospital-owned practices coalesce, they often defer decision making about privileges to the medical staff. Their assumption is that if the privileging process is good enough for the hospital, it is good enough for the group. While defaulting to the medical staff expedites the credentialing process, it becomes problematic over time for two reasons. First, from a quality perspective, medical staffs use no uniform benchmark other than the minimal standard of basic competence to ensure patient safety. Second, much of the work of the group practice takes place in ambulatory settings outside the purview of the organized medical staff.

The first issue raises the question of whether a hospital affiliated group practice should set its privileging standards higher than those to which other members of the medical staff are subject. While most medical staffs undertake their credentialing activities seriously and with appropriate diligence, their goal typically is to find a minimum threshold that indicates whether new and existing staff members are competent enough to exercise requested privileges. For open medical staffs, credentialing is meant to be an inclusive process that weeds out practitioners only if their abilities and skills are so deficient that they would put patients in danger. Most staffs are reluctant to disadvantage practitioners by limiting their scope of clinical activity. When this reluctance is combined with the ubiquitous fear of litigation that surrounds the healthcare environment today, we see the credentialing and reappointment processes devolve into *de facto* "permission to practice" unless there is a compelling reason to set limits on an individual.

Group practices have an opportunity to set expectations that have less to do with political compromise and more to do with strategic decisions related to quality goals. For instance, a group may decide to assign joint replacements to fellowship-trained orthopedists rather than generalists, even though medical staff policies are more inclusive. The group's standards cannot be less rigorous than those of the medical staff, but they can be more rigorous.

Second, the group needs to consider all of a physician's practice settings, whereas the hospital medical staff needs to consider practice only within the bricks and mortar of the institution (and at its secondary sites operating under formal hospital license, such as an ambulatory surgery center). Insurance carriers often mandate that all of their contracted physicians have hospital privileges, but the increasing utilization of hospitalists will progressively erode this convention. As a result of this trend, those with ambulatory practices (primary care physicians and many medical subspecialists) will be able to drop their hospital privileges and be exempt from the quality control mechanisms of the medical staff.

Given the limitations of a hospital-based credentialing process, the development of processes for credentialing all group members, regardless of practice setting, becomes incumbent on a new group practice.

Undertaking a group practice credentialing effort raises a host of new questions. What are the political consequences of having higher standards in the group? Do higher standards create increased liability for the group or its members? Are group practice members more likely to become subject to reports to the National Practitioner Data Bank if they fail to meet the group's higher privileging requirements? Will restricting the scope of practice of some members on the basis of the group's evolving privileging criteria cause damaging dissension and controversy among the group's physicians? What sort of management infrastructure will have to be added to implement a privileging program, and will it be cost-effective? Let's address each of these questions.

If the hospital affiliated group practice sets internal privileging standards higher than those set by the medical staff and hospital board, will there be political fallout? Invariably, the establishment of higher standards by the group practice will raise questions about the adequacy of the medical staff's standards. The medical staff credentials committee will be pressured to rethink its benchmarks and whether it should reset those bars to match the criteria of the group practice. Non–group members of the medical staff may feel threatened by the possibility of losing previously held privileges and may adopt a hostile posture toward the group. This animosity could affect referrals or make coexistence on the medical staff problematic. The group's leaders will have to weigh these concerns against the advantages of delivering superior care. These potential advantages include contribution to the group's reputation and market share, increased revenue under P4P formulas, decreased malpractice premiums, strengthened ability to recruit top-caliber physicians, and professional satisfaction.

Can the establishment of higher privileging standards in the group create liability for the organization? As with any policy, the group must adhere to the standards it adopts. Malpractice exposure is likely to decrease when a group adopts higher standards because they promote better clinical care. Liability increases only if standards are set but ignored.

If the group practice declines to grant a practitioner a privilege because it has higher standards than the medical staff, will this decision need to be reported to the National Practitioner Data Bank? The group analyzes and makes administrative decisions about its practitioners' capabilities to raise the quality of its output. A member's failure to meet the group's criteria for a particular scope of practice does not need to be reported to state authorities or the National Practitioner Data Bank.

Do privileging decisions have the potential to create dissension and controversy in the group? As with many of the decisions that the group practice will need to make as it develops and succeeds, this danger does exist. The best way to keep negativity in check is to provide effective guidance. Decision-making processes should be transparent, members should be well-educated on the issues and rationales for various decisions, and tactics should be justifiable by reference to the practice's mission and values. If privileging conflicts do arise, they should be resolved according to a clear policy on privileging disputes. Successful development of a culture committed to quality will dampen the frequency and intensity of such disagreements.

How does a group practice create an efficient infrastructure to support the tasks of credentialing and privileging? The initial step is to establish a committee to oversee the relevant activities. The group may want to include members who sit on the hospital's medical staff credentialing panel in this committee to import their training and experience in such matters. This overlap also helps the group practice committee avoid doing unnecessary work and research, as many of the policies adopted by the medical staff will also serve the group practice. The health system governing board should adopt policies that allow the two committees to share credentialing information. The careful background checks done by the hospital medical staff office should suffice for the group practice as well. In some cases, though, the group practice may wish to gather more information about a candidate than that acquired by the medical staff. For example, the medical staff may not be concerned about whether a candidate has a history of efficiency in an office setting, has a great bedside manner, or works well as a team member. The group practice credentials committee may want to explore such details to ensure the candidate is a strong fit for the group.

Vetting candidates for group membership is only one of the credentialing committee's tasks. Setting criteria that must be met to exercise privileges is another major undertaking. These privileging criteria may be identical to those granted by the hospital board to medical staff members or may be more rigorous. For example, the group practice may determine that only its fellowship-trained vascular surgeons will perform vascular surgery on its patients, even if general surgeons in the group hold hospital privileges to do this work, or it may determine that colonoscopies will be performed only by the group's gastroenterologists.

The group practice governing body may choose to step in at times to adjudicate privileges for political reasons. For example, if the practice needs to recruit a hand surgeon, the group practice board may feel it needs to steer all hand surgery to this position to attract such a specialist to the group. In this case, the restriction on other surgeons capable of performing hand surgery is not based on the quality of their work. When such a restriction is contemplated because some believe the specialist would deliver a higher level of care, the matter should go to the group practice credentials committee for exploration. This body should review the evidence-based literature, gather the insights of professional societies and recognized experts, take note of policies in highly regarded centers of excellence, and make a recommendation (along with the basis for that recommendation) to the practice governing body. If it recommends such restriction, the committee should forward to the board the criteria that should be used to qualify a practice member to exercise the privilege(s) in question.

The group practice credentials committee is also responsible for determining what procedures and activities should be permitted in its clinical space. The first time the group practice board learns that one of its members has been delivering controversial chelation therapy, for example, should not be when a malpractice suit is filed, a newspaper publicizes the fact, or a payer fraud unit makes inquiries. Clinical activities and procedures that are controversial or represent new technologies should require approval by the group's board after receipt of a recommendation from the credentials committee. The importance of this process will grow as more procedures move from the hospital into the outpatient arena and new office-based procedures are developed.

Building an effective process for credentialing and privileging in a group practice is an ambitious undertaking and generally does not begin until the group has established an infrastructure. If the group practice grows to encompass most of the hospital medical staff, the medical staff credentials function may then be delegated in its entirety to group practice management.

PEER REVIEW, RISK MANAGEMENT, UTILIZATION REVIEW, AND QUALITY IMPROVEMENT

Peer review is a fundamental element of medical education (e.g., mortality and morbidity conferences, grand rounds) and an accreditation requirement for hospital medical staffs. In most ambulatory settings, however, it is practiced only casually, and organizations rarely embed it in their approaches to quality improvement.

In the early stages of group development, hospital peer review activities are commonly assumed to be sufficient for uncovering quality concerns with practitioners. As the group grows in size and develops its own infrastructure, however, it will face an increasing need to extend the reach of sophisticated quality activities into ambulatory practice and should take the opportunity to create its own peer review processes designed to achieve a higher level of performance.

An early task for group practice leaders is to create an integrated approach to quality that includes peer review, risk management, utilization management, and quality improvement. Medical staff members commonly see these activities as separate from each other and as externally mandated matters of regulatory compliance. All too often, clinicians dismiss concerns about resource utilization as "something the bean counters worry about," while administrators focus on resource utilization (e.g., length of stay) as though it were the primary metric of success. When this polarization is at its worst, physicians perceive high quality and low resource utilization as incompatible. Payers and policy experts have stressed that this perspective misses the most critical point—the need for *value* in American medicine.[1]

The value advantage accruing to integrated delivery systems built around strong, established group practices has been studied and solidly documented. An article by Jay Sterns (2007) published in the *Journal of Health Care Finance* showed that 13 such organizations delivered care of comparable or better quality with fewer physician encounters, less hospital utilization, and lower ICU costs.

To be effective, efforts at improving clinical outcomes must be informed by a deep understanding of where, how, and why there are variations in care delivery.[2] Some of the best data about variations in care delivery stem from a focus on utilization. Group practices have an opportunity to sidestep the disconnection between utilization and quality that is prevalent in so many hospitals and redefine the ways quality and utilization are interrelated. (See Exhibit 11.1 for an example of how integration can facilitate quality improvement.) If a group practice has embraced a culture of quality and approaches its quality goals with rigor and diligence, peer review, risk management, and quality improvement become intrinsically driven rather than externally mandated.

Hospital affiliated group practices have access to considerably more performance data about their members than do typical small private practices in the community. The health system governing board should approve protocols that allow the hospital's medical staff and the group practice to share peer review information confidentially. The group practice quality committee should establish

---

Exhibit 11.1 Integrating Risk Management, Peer Review, Utilization Review, and Quality Improvement

Imagine that the hospital's utilization management department detects a trend of increasing ICU utilization, with longer stays and increased mortality. Preliminary analysis shows that patients with severe pulmonary diseases are so sick by the time they are admitted that they require longer stays. If quality and utilization are integrated, the following can happen immediately without cumbersome discussions or negotiation:

- The hospital's peer review process can shift to focused chart reviews of ICU patients.
- The hospital's risk management department can increase the sensitivity of its incident screening for ICU patients while the group's peer review activities can be directed toward the study of ambulatory treatment in key diagnostic groups before admission.
- The group's quality committee can engage its primary care providers and pulmonologists in the development of protocols that span ambulatory and inpatient care for pulmonary illnesses.
- The group's quality department can look for national programs and initiatives addressing the issues revealed by these activities.

---

performance monitors in settings not covered by the hospital's quality department. These data should be reviewed with the group's practicing physicians on an individual basis through periodic feedback reports. When potentially problematic performance trends are identified, the quality committee should engage practice leadership in fashioning and delivering appropriate interventions. As discussed in Chapter 8, this task is commonly delegated to the practice's medical director. However, it can be assigned to any practice leader who is likely to influence the practitioner involved.

These interventions should be collegial, reflecting the group's desire to help all of its members overcome clinical or behavioral deficiencies. The group should have clear policies on how to proceed, however, when collegial and supportive efforts don't improve the situation. When a situation involving serious quality concerns cannot be rectified, the group member(s) responsible for the deficiency should be asked to leave the group, either voluntarily or by way of the practice's termination procedures. The problem does not end there, however. Should the medical staff also investigate the physician's competence, which might lead, through legally mandated reporting criteria, to a data bank report on the physician in question?[3] Or should it avoid this endeavor and keep the reporting issue from surfacing? Can the medical staff investigate the activities of a member after he or she has resigned or been terminated?

Many hospital affiliated group practices have employment contracts with "co-terminus" provisions—that is, the practitioner agrees in the contract to voluntarily relinquish medical staff membership at the time employment is ended. Employment termination with automatic termination of medical staff membership is not necessarily a reportable event. If the employee was terminated as a result of incompetence or inappropriate behavior, however, the proper course of action is less clear. The group practice, medical staff, and hospital leaders should establish protocols for such issues before they arise.

PROTOCOL DEVELOPMENT AND DISEASE MANAGEMENT

Much has been written about the need for standardized approaches to common clinical conditions and for elimination of variation wherever it cannot be attributed to a unique patient need or justified by scientific evidence. Health policy experts, particularly those with a public health perspective, have been at the forefront of this push for evidence-based medicine (EBM). A convincing body of clinical evidence supports the use of standardized approaches to common conditions, as long as clinicians have discretion to depart from such guidelines in unique clinical situations. Nevertheless, the high value physicians place on autonomy has prompted many medical staffs to oppose this movement. Younger and more team-oriented physicians are generally more accepting of standardized clinical protocols than are some of their older peers.

Three attributes characterize group practices that have embraced protocol-driven treatment. First, evidence-based practice is a group norm. Strong group practices prioritize the endorsement of evidence- and consensus-based protocols. One or more quality committees typically provide this endorsement. In smaller groups, a quality subcommittee of the board often vets, recommends, and disseminates such protocols. In larger groups, multiple quality committees may be organized around service lines or clinical departments. These committees report to a central quality committee of the board to ensure that the service lines or departments are not adopting conflicting standards.

Second, members of protocol-driven groups work as one team across multiple sites of service. Enabling technology, especially a common EHR, is critical to these groups' uniformity. As primary care physicians migrate away from inpatient care, unitary treatment plans spanning ambulatory and acute care settings will become a distant memory unless practitioners see themselves as teammates developing an evidence-based treatment plan that crosses the spectrum of care delivery and accommodates unique patient needs.

Third, protocol-driven groups cluster patients with similar conditions and employ ancillary personnel (e.g., case managers, social workers, nutritionists) to provide them with education and support. Only through patient clustering can groups afford such interventions. For example, group education for diabetic patients has become increasingly popular. Doctors in solo practice may try to provide such education, but they can rarely afford to hire professionals such as teachers, social workers, nutritionists, and case managers to do this work. The group practice may find these services to be a cost-effective way to provide coordinated care for large groups of patients. Further, these professionals can provide group care that is consistent with clinical protocols as opposed to care that varies from one isolated doctor–patient encounter to another.

In group practices, the development of clinical protocols can be a professionally and intellectually rewarding activity. Clinicians should work together to select appropriate protocols, subject them to peer review, and measure local outcomes. Clinicians offered the opportunity to participate in protocol development will feel a greater sense of comfort and commitment than those who are simply told what to do. When commitment and buy-in are strong, group members speak about "our way of treating patients" with a sense of proprietary pride and excitement. Patients pick up on this sentiment and feel safer—confident that their physicians are committed to delivering coordinated and well-researched care.

Some group practices include physicians who enjoy creating new medical knowledge through the evaluation of performance data, assessment of outcomes resulting from the use of clinical protocols, or participation in research protocols. While the majority of group practices do not have formal academic ties, the presence of a large patient population often garners grant support from, or liaison with, nearby academic institutions, which enables the practice to engage in modest but interesting clinical research activities. Such activities promote ongoing learning and offer groups another opportunity to create a name for themselves.

PRACTICE PROFILING

The day-to-day pressures of patient care often distract clinicians from spotting trends in clinical management and responding appropriately. Group use of an EHR compensates for this oversight. From an EHR, a group's quality, case management, and utilization management staffs can acquire data—about the group as a whole as well as each practitioner—on any number of issues.

For instance, they can look at the number of diabetics in the entire panel of primary care patients; compare that figure to public health statistics to determine whether under-diagnosis may be occurring; look at the group's rates of screening for secondary morbidity, its rates of hospitalization, and its compliance with practice protocols; and set collective goals based on these data. They can then take a physician-by-physician look at the same issues, harnessing friendly internal competition to maximize protocol compliance or, where the data are available, to maximize outcomes. Screening and preventive measures that have been objectively validated, such as monitoring hemoglobin A1c in diabetes patients or providing vaccinations for children, should be areas of focus. The group practice culture should reduce or eliminate the physician resistance to profiling that is so prevalent on hospital medical staffs. Even in the best systems, adherence to guidelines is never 100 percent. By working toward that goal, groups exhibit behaviors that simultaneously benefit their patients and practice economics.

BEST PRACTICE IDENTIFICATION AND TRANSFER

Practice profiling leads us to another critical and differentiating feature of group practices—the ability to identify and quickly disseminate the best clinical practices. Given that translation of new knowledge into clinical practice takes a significant amount of time in the medical field, this matter is critical. A cultural commitment to adapting best practices, a compensation system that rewards practice improvement, and a leadership infrastructure that can disseminate lessons are key ingredients in this process.

This same approach to clinical best practice identification can be applied to other aspects of practice, including issues of cost and revenue, by making different comparisons:

- Which practice site has the highest rate of employee satisfaction? The highest rate of staff retention?
- Which site has the highest rate of patient satisfaction?
- Which cluster of physicians is most successful at minimizing cost per RVU generated?
- Which site has the highest percentage of copayment collection?

After identifying their most successful sites of service, group leaders can analyze how these sites generate their results (a kind of root cause analysis in reverse), and then disseminate these findings to other practice sites so that they, too, can maximize their effectiveness. They can also appoint physicians who have demonstrated impressive results as internal teachers or mentors. A physician struggling with a particular issue—for example, staff retention or patient throughput—can visit and shadow colleagues whose performance in these areas is exemplary. One clinic in the Midwest, for example, situates poorly organized or inefficient physicians next to efficient colleagues so they have ongoing exposure to better habits.

In addition to using quantitative data to identify best practices, multispecialty groups can harness the unique knowledge base of specialists to bolster primary care practice. See Exhibit 11.2.

TRACKING REFERRAL PATTERNS

The rate of *referral leakage*—sending patients outside the economic membrane of the group for clinical or diagnostic services—is important data and should be tracked by the group. While groups should have a legitimate quality argument for referring patients to their own practitioners—for example, they will provide the best care because they emphasize coordinated treatment, high credentialing standards, and a commitment to quality improvement—groups usually focus on their economic argument for referring internally. The economic argument is particularly compelling when the group receives capitated payments for patient care, but it also applies to other reimbursement models.

By tracking external referrals, leadership can monitor the loyalty and team spirit of the group's physicians, as well as systemic problems (e.g., gaps in the group's array of services, access problems, chronic dissatisfaction with a service). This task is not simple, however. Complex dynamics surface when a group expects its physicians to refer internally.

Exhibit 11.2 Camino Medical Group's Specialty Care/Primary Care Interface

For some years, the Camino Medical Group (now a part of the Palo Alto Foundation Medical Group) has had a tradition of holding regular teaching conferences in which a medical or surgical specialist updates the group's primary care practitioners (PCPs) on their particular specialty. As a result, PCPs are more confident treating more complex patients and the process of internal referral for specialty care is dramatically enriched.

(E. Lister, personal communication)

As hospital-owned groups coalesce, preexisting referral patterns will be disrupted. New recruits must understand the group's referral expectations and the rationale behind them. Otherwise, they will likely feel coerced and become embittered that they can no longer exercise autonomy in directing their patients' care.

On the other hand, the group may have strategic reasons to continue referring to certain non–group members. For instance, imagine that an established but independent group of high-quality orthopedists that has been loyal to the hospital for a long time participates in a lucrative, well-functioning ambulatory surgical center joint venture with the hospital. This group, for whatever reason, does not want to be employed. Even if the hospital affiliated group practice has orthopedists of its own, would turning patients away from this external group make sense? Strategic decisions about collaboration/competition need to be made carefully with system strategies and the economics of the entire enterprise in mind.

Finally, there are circumstances in which patient needs trump the group's referral preferences:

- Longstanding relationships between patients and specialists should not be disrupted unless patients request a transfer.
- Patient preference needs to be honored when preferences are strong and clear.
- Geographic considerations may be important when the group practice offers a service, but it is available only at a site significantly distant from the patient's location, and non-group, local referral options are available.
- If a group cannot meet a patient's clinical needs, the patient needs to be referred to sites that will most likely be able to address them.
- Physicians who are reluctant to refer internally because of doubts about a colleague's competence (clinical or behavioral) must bring the issue forward so leadership can resolve it. "Referring around" the clinician in question is not acceptable.

CONCLUSION: BACK TO EXPECTATIONS, EMPOWERMENT, AND ACCOUNTABILITY

Collectively, the practices described in this chapter offer enormous opportunities to improve care delivery. With regard to efficiency and effectiveness, they give group practices a chance of meeting healthcare purchasers' recurring demand for value. This set of practices is almost impossible to embed in a medical community of solo and small group providers working independently. With rare exceptions (such as an unusually effective independent practice association), only integrated systems working through a group practice provider network can effectively meet purchasers' expectations. To this end, the work of group formation, leadership, and culture building referenced earlier is essential. Clarifying expectations upon entry to the group, encouraging members to invent their own solutions to the challenges of practice, creating strong peer review and performance improvement programs to measure and assess care, and holding group members accountable are all essential activities and fundamental to sustaining the group practice advantage.

NOTES

1. *Value* is typically defined as quality divided by cost.

2. See the work of Jack Wennberg at www.dartmouthatlas.org.

3. When a medical staff and hospital board limit, restrict, or terminate a clinician's hospital privileges or medical staff membership on the basis of demonstrated incompetence or unprofessional conduct, this action must be reported to the federal National Practitioner Data Bank. Such a report must also be made if the practitioner resigns while under investigation by the medical staff. These procedures are mandated by the Health Care Quality Improvement Act, which can be accessed at www.npdb-hipdb.hrsa.gov/legislation/title4.html.

CHAPTER 12

Legal and Regulatory Concerns

HEALTHCARE TODAY is subject to significant legal and regulatory complexity. Hospitals must consider numerous legal and regulatory issues when they employ physicians and form group practices.

A detailed discussion of the legal issues presented in this chapter is beyond the scope of this book. The variation state statutes and local issues introduce makes a one-size-fits-all approach to legal matters imprudent; however, the issues identified in the following sections apply to any group practice development effort.

SEEK INFORMED LEGAL COUNSEL

Legal counsel should be consulted throughout a group development effort. Absent sound legal advice, hospitals can jeopardize their tax-exempt status, run afoul of anti-fraud/anti-kickback laws, become entangled in false claims litigation, incur huge fines, face the possibility of exclusion from Medicare and federal insurance programs, and even subject administrators to claims of criminal behavior. In addition, reputations can be indelibly tarnished, physician recruitment and retention efforts derailed, and institutional financial viability undermined.

Because healthcare regulations are complex and change constantly, administrators should seek legal counsel that specializes in health law. Reliance on local attorneys with limited experience may prompt unwelcome surprise visits from enforcement agencies. The principal professional organization for health law experts in the United States is the American Health Lawyers Association (www.ahla.org). Each year it conducts numerous educational programs, including the Physicians and Physician Organizations Law Institute and the Hospitals and Health Systems Law Institute.

Group practices may retain their own lawyer or rely on the firm or individuals retained by the hospital or health system. Independent counsel is germane only to practices that are separate corporate entities and have contractual relationships with hospitals. In such cases, to perform its fiduciary responsibilities properly, the board of the group practice needs legal input that is not conflicted by accountability to two parties. To keep the interests of the practice and the health system aligned, however, practice counsel should collaborate closely with hospital counsel.

For group practices that are divisions or subsidiaries of a health system and report to the system board, independent legal counsel is not warranted and may unnecessarily aggravate underlying tensions between group and hospital. (Differences between the group practice and the leadership of its parent organization should be handled through mechanisms other than legal channels whenever possible.)

DEVELOP THE STRUCTURAL RELATIONSHIP BETWEEN THE GROUP PRACTICE AND HOSPITAL/HEALTH SYSTEM

In the early planning stages, entities developing a clinical group need to determine where the practice will sit in the corporate organizational tree. Group placement and structure depend on numerous legal considerations, including tax matters, liability concerns, reporting relationships and accountability, antitrust factors, laws regulating the corporate practice of medicine, and other issues.

One approach is to organize the physician group as a subsidiary corporation with its own governance structure. A subsidiary is a corporation controlled by a "parent" organization that owns a majority of the corporation's stock and ensures that the corporation uses corporate funds properly and complies with corporate policies and procedures. The governing board of the parent corporation is responsible for keeping strategy aligned between the two corporations. Subsidiary corporations are used for many purposes, such as to limit the parent organization's liability for acts of the subsidiary.

When a subsidiary physician organization is formed, a decision must be made as to whether it will it be for profit or not for profit. If it is organized as a tax-exempt corporation, it must meet on its own merits the Internal Revenue Code's (IRC) requirements for exempt status. One advantage to forming a subsidiary physician corporation is that the hospital or health system retains strategic ownership but the subsidiary can allow for significant physician control over its operations, which can be carried out in a manner more consistent with that of successful physician office practices. At the same time, the subsidiary can take advantage of favorable contracts negotiated by the parent health system.

Another approach is to organize the employed group practice as a division within the health system, on a par with the system's hospital divisions. In this arrangement, hospitals and physicians report to the system governing board. This structure is easy to implement and involves little corporate restructuring other than the creation of clear reporting channels. Under this arrangement, the physician group practice division is not legally required to have its own practice board. Nevertheless, it would still be highly advisable to establish the equivalent of a board or executive committee for the group practice. As discussed in Chapter 7, physician "ownership" of the group practice enterprise—in a psychological sense—is imperative. The results described in this book are unlikely to be achieved unless a multispecialty group practice is governed by its physicians.

Some health systems establish a joint venture with physicians to create a home for the group practice. In this model, doctors and the health system share governance. Joint ventures are typically pursued when the parties share an interest in the bottom line of an enterprise (e.g., an ambulatory surgical or diagnostic center). Joint ventures are not as popular today as they were in the late 1990s and first years of the twenty-first century. As the physician population ages and many doctors approach retirement, they will have greater difficulty finding replacements to buy out their interests in these ventures. This projection diminishes the financial attractiveness of the joint venture to physician partners. Also, joint ventures with single-specialty groups are more likely to succeed than joint ventures with more complex multispecialty groups. As a structural model for hospital affiliated group practices, joint ventures are best used as bridging arrangements when full integration is not yet politically feasible in a medical community.

If the health system operates in a state that enforces prohibitions against the corporate practice of medicine (CPOM) (see the following section titled "Issues Related to the Corporate Practice of Medicine"), the contractual arrangement(s) affiliating the physician group and the health system have to be structured accordingly. For example, the group practice could be established as a clinic that affiliates with the health system, or it could be organized on the basis of a medical foundation model.

The extent of employed physicians' involvement in system governing boards must also be determined in not-for-profit arrangements. Historical rules of the Internal Revenue Service (IRS) have allowed "interested persons" to compose up to 49 percent of board membership. *Interested persons* are employees such as the hospital/health system CEO and physicians who treat patients in, do business with, or derive financial benefit from the organization. In general, the practice of placing employees on the governing board of not-for-profit institutions has been discouraged. Limiting the number of employees who may sit on the board is prudent, particularly on boards that establish the salaries of employed physicians. However, many organizations are seeking to give such physicians greater leadership roles in their health systems. With this goal in mind, legal counsel should be consulted to determine whether and how many employed group practice physicians can sit on various boards in the health system. In many cases, organizations will want to take note of the safe-harbor requirements of IRC section 4958 regarding intermediate sanctions that encourage establishment of an independent committee or independent boards of directors (that do not have conflicts of interest) to make compensation decisions.

An issue that sometimes surprises and distresses physicians elected or appointed to a hospital or health system board is the requirement for public disclosure of their salary. Not-for-profit hospitals must file Form 990 with the IRS so it can monitor for unreasonable salaries and benefits. These documents are often accessed by local newspapers and disseminated annually in print and online. While high-level hospital administrators may be accustomed to this exposure, doctors who have come from the private practice world are not. This requirement should be discussed with employed physicians who will be joining health system boards so they do not feel sandbagged when the Form 990 is released.

ISSUES RELATED TO THE CORPORATE PRACTICE OF MEDICINE

Prohibition of CPOM originated with the medical profession in the early 1900s and still continues in some states. The underlying purpose of these statutes was to bar non-licensed laypersons and businesses from interfering with the medical judgment of licensed physicians. Courts generally accept this ethical restriction as a matter of public policy. Over half of the states recognize this doctrine, either statutorily or as common law. Nevertheless, most have done little to enforce the doctrine, and it is generally seen as hostile to contemporary approaches to healthcare delivery, including the development of integrated delivery systems.

Today, all states have passed laws enabling physicians to incorporate their practices. CPOM laws, however, can prohibit hospitals from employing physicians. California and Texas are the most notable states enforcing this restriction.[1] Hospitals are advised to explore the CPOM laws of the state in which a hospital affiliated group practice is planned and the degree to which they are enforced.[2]

In states that prohibit physician employment, typically one or more legal "workarounds" enable hospitals to create or contract with affiliated physician groups. These workarounds usually involve some version of "the Foundation Model." This arrangement is built around a medical foundation—a not-for-profit body that may control one or more hospitals and contracts with payers to provide clinical services to insured patients. Under this model, the foundation enters into a contract with a group practice to be its exclusive provider of medical care within a geographic or specialty service area. This contract, called a professional services agreement (PSA), sends a payment stream to the group practice. The foundation usually employs the entire front and back office support staff of the group practice, freeing the group from administrative burdens. Medical foundations are often instrumental in facilitating the development of the group practices with which they associate.

ACCREDITATION CONCERNS

To participate in Medicare/Medicaid programs, hospitals must comply with federal Conditions of Participation. Most institutions meet this requirement through accreditation by The Joint Commission, the Healthcare Facilities Accreditation Program, or DNV (Det Norske Veritas). Hospitals that have traditionally focused accreditation readiness on inpatient services will need to understand and address the requirements accrediting agencies have for hospital-owned physician practices. Physicians accustomed running their own private practices will need to understand that, as part of a hospital or health system, their new practice environment may be subject to the ambulatory requirements of the hospital's accrediting organization. Significant compliance failures by the hospital affiliated group practice can put the entire institution's accreditation status at risk.

Standards for ambulatory practice are also promulgated by organizations other than those granted deemed status to accredit on behalf of the Centers for Medicare & Medicaid Services (CMS). Use of these organizations is typically voluntary but may strengthen the operations and reputation of the affiliated group practice. Examples include the Accreditation Association for Ambulatory Health Care, National Committee for Quality Assurance, URAC, and American Association for Accreditation of Ambulatory Surgery Facilities. In addition, some states have imposed their own regulations on hospital outpatient endeavors and ambulatory practices. Hospital and physician leaders need to consider the best ways to comply with requirements and whether to participate in voluntary accreditation programs.

Although it is not an accreditation organization, the professional association for large physician group practices is the American Medical Group Association (AMGA) (www.amga.org). AMGA activities provide opportunities to network and pool collective wisdom about the challenges of running large group practices.

COMPENSATION CONCERNS

An array of federal and state laws and regulations affect the form physician compensation takes and the amount paid. The following factors have a legal impact on compensation arrangements: the source of the compensation funds, the tax status of the organization(s) involved, the nature of the physician relationship (e.g., ownership, contractual, or employment), and whether payments are made directly or indirectly. Legal and accounting advice should be sought when setting up a group practice compensation structure.

In general, legal concerns regarding compensation aggregate around two bodies of laws: IRC and laws to which tax-exempt organizations are subject; and laws that govern federal health programs, particularly the Stark self-referral laws and the federal anti-kickback statutes. Legal counsel should always review any compensation arrangements being proposed for use by the hospital affiliated group practice. While significant attention must be paid to federal legal constraints, local laws should not be overlooked. For example, many states have their own anti-kickback statutes and "mini-Stark" laws.

Tax-Exempt Status and Prohibited Inurement

Not-for-profit hospitals must be careful not to improperly transfer "community" funds to private individuals. *Private inurement* occurs when a nonprofit health system's assets or earnings are used for the benefit of an individual rather than for the organization. One example is when an individual receives benefits from the health system/hospital that are greater than those he or she provides in return. The most common type of private inurement is excessive compensation, and care must be taken that employed physicians in a hospital affiliated group practice are paid salaries that reflect market realities. If a *for-profit* healthcare corporation pays unreasonable compensation to an employee, the excess amount will be deemed a taxable distribution to the employee and the corporation will be denied a compensation deduction of the excess amount. For a *tax-exempt* healthcare entity, the excess amount of compensation is considered an asset that the organization has *inured* to a private individual in violation of IRC section 501(c)(3).

The federal government can revoke an organization's tax-exempt status if it has engaged in private inurement. The IRS monitors non-profit organizations and can impose intermediate sanctions for paying unreasonable salaries and benefits. Board members can face significant tax and legal exposure under IRC section 4958 if they authorize excessive compensation.[3] In recent years, the IRS has become more tuned in to the various benefits that may be directed to physicians working for hospitals, which it sometimes considers an expropriation of community funds. Care must be taken when physicians are compensated for serving as a service line medical director, participating in the emergency department call schedule, assuming the administrative duties of a department chair, or other such tasks. In all cases, the compensation amount should be based on market norms, and there should be evidence that real and valuable work is being performed in exchange for the payment.

The federal government periodically advises hospitals on how to calculate fair market value, but hospitals and their group practices should always seek expert guidance on approved methodologies before undertaking a fair market value analysis.

Navigating the Minefield of Stark Regulations and Anti-Kickback Statutes

The Stark laws, sometimes known as the physician self-referral laws, have been evolving for nearly two decades. The essence of these laws is a prohibition on physician referrals for certain designated health services (DHS) to entities with which the doctor has an ownership and/or compensation arrangement. Entities that provide DHS to a patient as a result of a tainted referral are also prohibited from billing for those services.

In 2007 and 2008, a flurry of new rules and changes took place in the Stark regulatory field. In this same period, the federal government stepped up its enforcement of these laws. As this book goes to press, it appears that CMS will soon be requiring that, to ensure compliance with the latest iteration of Stark regulations, all Medicare-participating hospitals submit comprehensive reports that describe their financial relationships with physicians. On September 5, 2007, CMS issued "final" regulations on the Stark laws—the third of three phases, referred to as *Phase III regulations*. In-depth discussion of the Stark regulations is beyond the scope of this book, but readers are encouraged to further their understanding of these laws through the many resources available on the subject.[4]

The Stark laws are *strict liability* laws, which means that a physician who has a financial relationship with any entity implicated by the law is prohibited from making referrals to that entity for DHS unless an exception applies. Intent and awareness of the violation are irrelevant—any violation can result in penalties.

Conversely, the federal anti-kickback statutes require that there be intent and knowledge of the violation for penalties to be imposed. These statutes generally prohibit the offer, solicitation, or payment of any remuneration in exchange for a patient referral when the services to be delivered will be paid for by a federal health insurance program. Since so many relationships between doctors and hospitals can be implicated under these laws, *safe-harbor* provisions have been promulgated to provide legal exceptions. A number of safe harbors apply to physician compensation models, including those that apply to bona fide employment arrangements and personal service and management contracts. Most important in any situation is for compensation for physician services to be generally consistent with the fair market value of those services, without any financial remuneration based on the physician's referral patterns. Hospital affiliated group practices must take great care if they establish a system that considers system-wide performance in their physician compensation arrangements. Such arrangements can exist, but close legal attention is necessary to ensure they are compliant with the various anti-kickback statutes.

The rise of P4P incentives is a trend that is creating new legal questions. In late 2008, the Office of Inspector General (OIG) indicated that it will allow a hospital and a physician group to share the financial incentives the hospital receives when it meets a payer's P4P targets. They cannot do so, however, until strict OIG rules have been met.

Beyond the laws discussed here, compensation for group practice physicians is subject to many other statutes, regulations, and rules, including state and federal laws governing payroll deduction, employee benefits, retirement plans, and deferred compensation arrangements. Hospitals' human resources departments can be an excellent source of information regarding the issues involved.

CONFLICT OF INTEREST CONCERNS

Health system, hospital, and group practice leaders should identify all circumstances in which significant or potential conflict exists. Traditional conflict of interest policies address circumstances in which board members or other organizational decision makers might be predisposed to act in ways that are not in the best interests of the institution. In this regard, the group practice governing board should adopt and enforce a clear conflict of interest policy.

Conflict of interest should also be addressed in the recruitment and employment policies of the physician practice. For example, should a group practice member be allowed to invest in a competing diagnostic or treatment facility? Some community physicians seeking to join the hospital affiliated group practice may already have such investments and may wish to retain them. Adoption of an explicit conflict of interest policy will clarify whether they are permissible. It should not only alert doctors seeking to join the group, but also lay out for incumbents the consequences (if any) of making such investments.

Dual employment is another potential conflict of interest. A physician may want to work part time for another hospital or group practice. For example, a shift work emergency physician may decide to moonlight on his or her days off. Conflict of interest policies should clearly indicate whether such arrangements are permissible. They should also address concerns about how dual income streams will affect compensation from the group practice. Where should funds go that are generated by group practice members for speaking engagements, enrollment of their patients in research protocols, drug trial fees, and so forth? Do these dollars get pooled into the general revenues of the group practice, or are they assignable to an individual physician? Once again, it is important to have clear policies that indicate what revenue sources are considered acceptable and how revenue streams will be directed.

Conflicts of interest can be addressed in employment contracts, but conflict of interest policies are useful because they can be modified as necessary and applied to all physicians in the group, eliminating the need to change individual contracts.

Conflicts of interest regarding practice members' ties to medical device makers, pharmaceutical companies, and other commercial enterprises have been drawing significant amounts of public attention in the past few years. Visits from pharmaceutical personnel have become a practice that diminishes the credibility of the medical profession in the eyes of the public. Some professional organizations are passing codes of conduct outlining strict parameters for physician–industry relationships. In addition, some legislative bodies have been placing restrictions on these practices. Where industry–physician interaction has been extensive and dollars have been exchanged, fraud investigations have become more frequent. Health system and group practice leaders should explore the ethical, professional, and legal implications of these conflicts and adopt and communicate clear policies on this controversial topic. One prominent physician group practice among the first to establish such policies is the Cleveland Clinic.

Group practices that engage in industry-supported research protocols need to be particularly cognizant of potential conflicts and may wish to avoid even the appearance of impropriety. The group practice may wish to adopt conflict of interest policies that parallel those of the hospital or invoke more stringent guidelines. A group practice that does extensive research may even want to establish its own institutional review board.

EMPLOYEE OR MEMBER OF THE MEDICAL STAFF? A MAZE OF ISSUES

Many or all of the physicians in the group practice are likely to be members of the hospital/health system's medical staff. Practicing as both an employee and a medical staff member can raise issues that have legal implications. Therefore, it is important to note that not all group practice members may need to join the medical staff. Those that practice exclusively in the outpatient arena, for example, may have no compelling reason to do so.

Medical staff membership by group practice physicians raises a number of issues. For example, organized medical staff members are sometimes eligible to receive stipends to perform medical staff work (e.g., serving as a medical staff officer, taking emergency call, or serving as a department chair). Should group practice members employed by the hospital be eligible for such payments, or should compensation for this work be considered part of their employment agreement? If a physician is receiving two payment streams, might they amount to compensation beyond fair market value, thereby raising red flags regarding private inurement and anti-kickback statutes?

Performance deficiencies pose yet another dilemma. Should such problems be handled as employment issues or medical staff issues? Group practice physicians may insist that their clinical and behavioral deficiencies be handled by the medical staff because most medical staff bylaws guarantee extensive due process in determining whether corrective action is warranted. Handling a physician performance concern as an employment issue may deprive the doctor of the checks and balances available through these bylaws.

Consequences of deficient or unprofessional performance must be addressed in the contracts of employed physicians. Are the performance concerns an adequate "for cause" basis for termination? Is a grievance procedure outlined or referred to in the contract? Are medical staff due process rights considered waived if termination occurs under the contract? Will the group practice subsidize remedial education? Will leaves of absence for remedial education or participation in impaired physician programs be permissible? If yes, how will they be managed? These questions pose just a few of the decisions that need to be spelled out in contractual arrangements with group practice doctors.

A related concern is confidential information sharing. Should medical staff peer review data be available to group practice leaders? Should performance data generated by the group practice be shared with medical staff peer review committees? Again, the hospital and group practice must adopt clear policies on peer review information sharing so that there are no unsanctioned breaches of confidentiality. Competent counsel can be helpful in drawing up the requisite policies. Such policies should address credentialing as well as peer review data.

Over time, if the composition of the medical staff becomes identical to the membership of the group practice (or almost identical), restructuring or reassignment of responsibilities may be necessary. Are both organizations needed? Can all medical staff functions be performed by the group practice? Why, for example, should credentialing or quality monitoring be carried out by two organizations if one will suffice?

Most hospitals today have medical staff structures that were designed in the early days of the last century. The growth of a group practice provides an opportunity to revise the traditional roles of the organized medical staff. Health system boards may even consider delegating medical staff functions exclusively to its group practice. Before undertaking a creative restructuring of this sort, thoughtful legal counsel should be sought.

CORPORATE COMPLIANCE ACTIVITIES

Enforcement of healthcare regulations and compliance requirements has intensified in the past few years. Most healthcare organizations have responded by strengthening their internal compliance programs. A hospital affiliated group practice presents many opportunities to inadvertently run afoul of the complex web of regulatory requirements and, for this reason, should be brought under the purview of the hospital's compliance program. Some practices become large enough that they can justify appointing their own internal compliance officer. Regardless of how compliance oversight is structured, it must be adequate enough to protect the institution, including its group practice physicians, from enforcement action by OIG and other regulatory enforcement agencies. As noted elsewhere in this chapter, these agencies have become particularly interested in financial relationships between hospitals and doctors and are monitoring them with great scrutiny. Compliance officers must closely monitor the evolving interpretations of regulations and update the hospital and group practice boards regularly on issues of potential concern.

In addition to the financial arrangements between the hospital/health system and doctors, the most critical concern from a compliance standpoint is coding and billing practice. Questionable coding and billing by doctors in small private practices may fly under the radar of enforcement agencies. In large group practices they are much less likely to do so. Physicians may need extensive training and oversight to break antiquated coding habits and comply with the policies and procedures of the group practice. Routine audits will identify physicians whose practices are out of line. In such cases, practice leaders should intervene promptly.

Groups are advised to consider establishing a regular education and training program geared toward achieving regulatory compliance. Many physicians will resist spending time on nonclinical education, so leaders should impress upon their colleagues the influence good compliance practices (or lack thereof) can have on the practice's reputation, financial viability, and long-term durability.

GOVERNING DOCUMENTS, POLICIES, AND PROCEDURES

If the group practice is a self-governing entity, it should have a set of bylaws that articulate its governing principles and its approach to internal management. Consistency of group bylaws with those of the hospital or health system is important. These bylaws should be written clearly, with minimum legal jargon. In these increasingly volatile times, bylaws should be flexible so they can be amended with relative ease to accommodate the ongoing evolution of the group practice and health system. Bylaws typically contain clauses that outline the duties of the board of directors; the number and term of office of board members, along with qualifications for eligibility; the officers of the organization; and standing committees of the board.

In addition to bylaws, the group practice should develop comprehensive policies and procedures that spell out the manner in which day-to-day operations of the group will be performed. Since the members of the new group practice will have come from disparate practice settings, the group needs to have clear policies that establish the uniform approaches expected in their new practice home.

Many of these group practice policies deal with matters that are potentially problematic under federal and state laws, such as professional conduct (e.g., sexual harassment), recordkeeping requirements, confidentiality and maintenance of privacy in accordance with HIPAA, informed consents, and coding and billing. Sample documents and compendiums of policies can be found in the online bookstores of organizations such as the American Group Management Association and the Medical Group Management Association.

RECRUITMENT AND PRACTICE ACQUISITIONS

Most hospital affiliated group practices will have an ongoing need to expand, which can be achieved through recruitment of individual doctors or by approaching the members of private physician practices in the area. Unlike hospital practice acquisitions of the 1980s and 1990s, few hospitals today offer goodwill payments for physician practices. However, whether a hospital pays for hard assets only or makes an offer for goodwill, it is critical to do a fair market valuation of what will be purchased. Failure to do so can trigger concerns about private inurement and raise suspicions under the anti-kickback laws regarding the possible purchase of referrals.

When recruiting new physicians to a hospital affiliated group practice, consideration must be paid to the Stark regulations described earlier, which were updated in 2007 (Stark III). Great care must be paid to the types of assistance that are used to facilitate recruitment. The Stark regulations have extensive provisions that are meant to distinguish permissible from impermissible tactics for attracting physicians to an organization. In general, the law has a physician recruitment exception that permits remuneration from a hospital to recruit a physician to relocate to that hospital's geographic area and join its staff. However, certain criteria must be met, including: (1) the agreement is in writing and signed by both parties; (2) the arrangement is not conditioned on the recruited physician referring patients to the hospital; and 3) the remuneration is not based on the number of referrals from the recruited physician. Additional recruitment restrictions imposed by the Stark regulations are extensive, and the parameters of a hospital recruitment effort should always be guided by knowledgeable counsel.

In designing employment contracts for new recruits, it is important to recognize the fluid nature of emerging strategies for hospital–physician alignment. Long-term contracts may lock in terms that are not sustainable, run afoul of changing regulatory constraints, create dissension within an emerging group practice leadership team, or be inconsistent with a compensation formula adopted by a maturing group practice. Consideration should be given to contract language that facilitates renegotiation and avoids long-term commitments. Sometimes employment contracts grant exclusive access to particular hospital service lines (often referred to as *exclusive contracts*). In such cases, it is important that the contract be a result of a careful medical staff "manpower" assessment, and only after the hospital or health system board has made an "on the record" determination that such exclusivity is in the best interests of the community. Group cohesion is advanced by creating consistent contracts with consistent terms; significant variability in employment contracts is apt to stimulate concerns about unfairness.

RESTRICTIVE COVENANTS

Private-practice physician groups commonly include restrictive covenants in their contracts. Under a restrictive covenant, a physician agrees not to participate in a competing practice following termination of employment with the group. Groups subject their doctors to these terms to prevent them from "using" the group to establish a community presence and then joining a competitor. Competitors may include practices owned by other hospitals, managed care companies, private practitioners, and physician management companies.

Restrictive covenants are commonly described as "noncompete" agreements. The enforcement of restrictive covenants varies by jurisdiction. They are most viable when written for limited periods (e.g., the restriction applies for no more than two years) and when the geographic area they cover is not overly expansive. Local legal counsel should be knowledgeable about local courts' likelihood to enforce noncompete agreements.

Despite the risk of competition, most hospital affiliated practices choose not to impose restrictive covenants in their employment agreements. Physicians dislike being subject to these clauses, and practices that impose them may have difficulty attracting prospective employees. Doctors want to be able to resume private practice if the employment experience does not work out—an option they do not have locally under a restrictive covenant. To allow physicians this safety net, some group practices write noncompete clauses that bar future employment with institutional competitors of the health system only (i.e., another hospital or health system seeking expansion in the service area).

ANTITRUST CONCERNS

When health systems grow through employment of physicians and acquisition of local practices, regulators may perceive their dominance of the physician community as having an anticompetitive effect in the marketplace. State and federal antitrust laws apply to healthcare providers, and government regulators appear to be watching marketplace consolidation closely. Historically, the Justice Department and the Federal Trade Commission have vigorously supported competition among healthcare providers. They view their mission as keeping healthcare markets free from restraints that hinder growth and development of new and innovative forms of competition. These agencies primarily work under three powerful federal statutes: The Sherman Act (sections 1 and 2); the Clayton Act (as amended by the Robinson-Patman Act); and the Federal Trade Commission Act. Antitrust regulation is a complex field, and once again, specialized legal counsel should be sought when guidance is needed.

CONCLUSION

As with any endeavor in healthcare today, physician group practice formation is subject to labyrinthine legal complexities. To avoid serious adverse legal consequences, knowledgeable legal counsel should be engaged before moving forward with hospital–physician alignment. A checklist of steps that should trigger consideration of legal options can be found in Exhibit 12.1. When carefully guided, a hospital affiliated group practice is not only an attractive option for physicians, but a legally permissible pathway to greater integration across a healthcare system.

Exhibit 12.1 Checklist of Legal/Regulatory Issues and Practices for Hospital Affiliated Group Practices

1. Engage knowledgeable health counsel.
2. Create an organizational structure that appropriately places the physician practice and its members within the hospital or health system.
3. Understand your local laws on corporate practice of medicine and determine whether they are enforced.
4. Create compensation structures that comply with the Internal Revenue Code, the Stark laws, and anti-kickback statutes.
5. Create a corporate compliance function for the group.
6. Determine the relationship between medical staff status and employment status of group physicians.
7. Comply with Stark and other legal restrictions on physician recruitment and practice acquisition.
8. Understand the antitrust implications of physician practice consolidation and expanding hospital–physician integration.
9. Create employment contract terms that address termination and its impact on medical staff status, whether restrictive covenants will be imposed, due process and grievance rights, and other considerations discussed in this chapter.
10. Create appropriate governing documents (e.g., bylaws, rules, procedures, policies).
11. Establish clear conflict of interest policies.
12. Be cognizant of accreditation requirements and their impact on the group practice and hospital/health system.

NOTES

1. For a list of state positions, see "Corporate Practice of Medicine Doctrine: A 50-State Survey Summary" at www.capc.org/tools-for-palliative-care-programs/hospital-hospice-tools/corporate-practice.pdf.

2. For example, the Medical Board of California discusses CPOM at www.medbd.ca.gov/licensee/corporate_practice.html.

3. IRC section 4958 deals with intermediate sanctions and notes that an "excess

benefit transaction" is any "non-fair market value" exchange benefiting a dis-
qualified person.

4. One example of such material is *Stark Final Regulations: A Comprehensive Analysis of Key Issues and Practical Guide*, 4th edition, by Charles B. Oppenheim, Esq., published in 2008 by the American Health Lawyers Association.

PART IV

CHAPTER 13

From Integrated Group to Integrated System

PREVIOUS CHAPTERS OF THIS BOOK have focused on the creation of a group practice and the establishment of its infrastructure. A well-functioning group practice provides a level of service, quality, and efficiency that can advance hospital and health system goals. Cohesive groups can go further to change the nature of their employer institution by strengthening hospital operations and assuming an increasing role in system leadership.

GROUP ASSIMILATION OF HOSPITAL-BASED SERVICES

In the first wave of physician employment, hospitals began by hiring primary care providers. These days, employed surgical specialists are just as likely to be recruited from the start. Whether primary care providers or specialists form the core of the group, most practices will want to expand to include the hospital-based clinical practitioners who deliver critical services, such as hospitalists and emergency room physicians; pulmonologists and critical care practitioners; and radiologists, anesthesiologists, and pathologists.

There are two major advantages to adding these traditionally hospital-based physicians to the group practice. First, the group's commitment to collegiality and collaboration enhances the seamlessness of care delivery when these hospital services are provided by group physicians. As a result, patient satisfaction should improve, lengths of hospital stay should shorten, resource utilization should become more predictable, and handoffs during patient admission and discharge should become more effective. Second, these assimilated clinical departments can influence the care delivery patterns of practitioners who are not affiliated with the group by applying the group's standardized protocols and best practices, articulating uniform expectations, exercising peer authority, and modeling collaborative behavior.

Despite the advantages assimilation promises, certain physician behaviors will inevitably introduce obstacles to integration. For example, a significant percentage of hospitalists, emergency room physicians, and other hospital-based specialists have developed a "shift work" approach to care delivery. In some areas of the country, physicians often fly into town for several shifts and then fly home. In terms of technical competence of care delivered, this model can produce quality results, but it does not provide an integrated approach to care delivery.

Many physicians working in these specialties have preferentially aligned with single-specialty groups in their discipline, including large single-specialty groups that serve many hospitals and span extensive geographies. Enticing these practitioners to move to a multispecialty group can be a challenge.

THE CHALLENGE OF MAINTAINING ALIGNMENT WITH INDEPENDENT PHYSICIANS

A daunting obstacle to group practice growth involves maintaining optimal engagement and alignment with independent physicians on the medical staff. The early chapters of this book described physicians as members of a beleaguered profession who are not inclined toward institutional loyalty. Their attitude toward competition, however, is a different story. Physicians tend to be competitive and are alert to being disadvantaged by an uneven playing field. When hospitals appear to favor one group—employed physicians—and invest significant resources in the evolution and success of that group, they should not be surprised when independent physicians cry foul.

Hospitals and health systems, dependent on referrals from independent as well as affiliated physicians, are understandably sensitive to these protests. Hospital CEOs and boards are forced to make a difficult choice—to either attenuate efforts at group formation or find some way to modulate the protests of independent physicians. Whenever possible, the latter is the better choice. An effective way of modulating independent doctors' protests is to provide even-handed support of *any* physician whose clinical practice, business model, and quality metrics contribute to hospital success. The Stark laws and other legal obstacles significantly limit the extent to which this support can be provided, but within those limits, equity and fairness need to dictate hospital practice. Physicians prepared to honor the covenants of group membership should be invited into the group. Physicians who prefer independent practice or who do not have the temperament to thrive in a group need to be appreciated for the value they bring to the hospital.

To keep independent physicians aligned with the hospital's interests, the group may need to voluntarily sacrifice some of its income stream and support these physicians by referring patients to them from time to time or by deciding not to hire certain specialists (e.g., "Dr. X is not a member of the group but is the best hand surgeon in the region. He collaborates well with us. While he doesn't want to join the group, he can still be 'our' hand surgeon."). This kind of cooperative, noncompetitive outreach can be powerful in mitigating tension between group and non-group doctors. Nevertheless, the costs and benefits of this approach need to be kept in mind. When a business case for supporting independent practice cannot be made, efforts at recruiting non-group doctors into the group need to intensify.

GROUP PARTICIPATION IN HOSPITAL LEADERSHIP

Leadership of an acute care hospital is a complex matter, involving not only a management team with a set of direct reporting relationships to the CEO, but also a medical staff leadership structure, and often a number of appointed physician leaders (for example, a vice president of medical affairs and medical directors of clinical services and programs).

The more the group practice develops physician leaders, the more it becomes an ideal setting from which to select medical directors. The skills cultivated in the group practice setting—communication, inclusion, and collaborative problem solving—all translate well to the hospital environment.

The process of appointing hospital medical directors should be nonpolitical and emphasize the responsibilities and accountabilities of the job. When clear criteria are established—including skills, competencies, and alignment with the hospital's mission, strategies, and goals—selection of physician leaders is straightforward and credible. If group members become represented disproportionately in the leadership ranks, this majority presence will not be attributable to just group membership; group members may meet the criteria more often than independent physicians do because of the group's investment in their training. Transparency about this process dampens independent physicians' suspicions of bias. If non–group members meet the criteria, they too can play a useful leadership role and deserve to be appointed.

The Use of Operating Councils

To increase physician engagement and improve efficiency, some hospitals are creating operating councils, which bring practicing physicians into small work groups with senior managers for the purpose of strengthening a service line. These groups collaboratively set operating agendas and oversee improvement initiatives. Operating councils are most effective when they target specific, critical functional areas in the hospital (the operating room, for instance) and involve only physicians seriously committed to improving the functional area in question. The *initial* work of such councils should be to make the service line more user-friendly for doctors who see a large number of patients. This agenda ensures physician buy-in to the broader revenue enhancement and performance improvement goals of the operating council. Physicians should be appointed rather than elected to serve on these councils and, ideally, should represent multiple disciplines. As noted for medical directors in the previous section, leaders cultivated in the group practice environment are natural candidates for operating council membership but should not be the only physicians considered. Commitment, alignment, and service line familiarity are key criteria for selection.

Through medical directorships and participation on operating councils, group leaders help coordinate care delivery across the acute care/ambulatory care boundary, foster physician/administrative partnership, bring clinical insights to the redesign of care delivery, and model collaborative approaches to clinical practice for their independent physician colleagues.

Medical Staff Leadership

The model of the organized medical staff that originated in the early part of the last century is becoming increasingly irrelevant to the work of most physicians and is often a barrier to hospitals in their pursuit of strategic success, but outdated Medicare Conditions of Participation and accreditation requirements are keeping it on life support. Obsolescence of the organized medical staff will be accelerated by the growth of strong, well-developed group practices that can provide the physician expertise and leadership lacking in many traditional medical staff organizations. Hospitals that have large group practices should discourage the organized medical staff from engaging in activities other than participation in the required tasks of peer review and credentialing. Where possible, the medical staff should be encouraged to downsize its infrastructure, and the hospital should appoint physicians with appropriate talent to address other leadership needs. As indicated in previous discussion, this talent can be drawn from both independent and employed or contracted physician pools. In addition, members of the group practice should actively participate in medical staff credentialing and peer review. As long as the traditional medical staff structure persists, group practice leaders should regularly run for medical staff officer and executive committee positions. The increase of hospital-employed physicians has caused some independent medical staff members to advocate bylaws that restrict group practice members' citizenship rights. These doctors view the medical staff as a bastion from which to oppose the ongoing transformation of medical care, particularly the physician employment trends sweeping the United States. Health system governing boards must watch for such amendment proposals and should not approve these ill-advised changes.

GROUP PARTICIPATION IN HOSPITAL/HEALTH SYSTEM GOVERNANCE

Recent surveys suggest that physicians constitute 20 to 40 percent of most hospital/health system boards. However, given that conflicts of interest will inevitably surface, there has been debate over whether employed physicians should be board members. For the most part, experts argue that all practicing physicians have conflicts of some sort and that the benefit of including engaged physicians on the board overshadows concerns about employment and independence. They also suggest that physician board members (other than the elected chief of staff) be selected through the same process that governs the selection of all other directors—against a set of explicit criteria.

As a hospital's employed group grows in size and strategic importance, the board should be selectively populated with members of the employed group. By sitting on the board, these physicians will develop a deeper sense of responsibility for the hospital/system's mission and goals. As stewards of the entire enterprise, they will be forced to think of the big picture and will take that perspective back to the group. Bringing this comprehensive vision to the group's culture will help modulate its natural tendency to become physician-centric. The presence of group members on the board also emphasizes the importance of looking beyond hospital operations to care delivery across the continuum. This more complex perspective is more likely to produce sustainable care delivery and business success.

CLOSED OR OPEN MEDICAL STAFF?

As the group becomes an increasingly dominant source of admissions and referrals and independent physicians' strategic significance fades, questions naturally emerge about whether to close the medical staff to non–group members and make the hospital the exclusive province of the group. While the hospital may benefit from improved control and standardization of the care delivery process, restricting membership of the medical staff should not even be considered until the group practice can meet the gamut of patient needs and handle over 90 percent of hospital admissions. Even under these circumstances, there is little to be gained by closing the staff if the group practice already dominates hospital activity and non–group members have become sufficiently aligned with the hospital's mission.

Instead of closing the entire medical staff, the hospital can take other steps to help the group practice set a high bar for physician performance. For example, the hospital can eliminate exclusive contracts with non-group providers of hospital-based services and direct those services to the group. Alternatively, the hospital can assign management of exclusive contracts to the group, which would hold practitioners under those contracts to appropriate performance standards. The hospital also can restrict the providers eligible to deliver high-acuity services (e.g., intensive care, neonatal intensive care, bariatric surgery, cardiothoracic surgery) and make the group the sole provider in these clinical areas. As another option, the hospital can adopt a policy that requires all medical directors to be group practice members.

WHEN, IF EVER, DOES THE GROUP EVOLVE TO LEAD THE SYSTEM?

Although physicians know a great deal about medical care delivery, they sometimes are not aware of the knowledge they lack about running complex health systems. For this reason, senior health system leaders need to guide and coach the leaders of a growing group practice so they acquire a deep understanding of the organization's role as a community resource and the management and operations of a health system. They also must learn to be accountable for community needs and not just those of their patients. Group physicians who are interested in more complex leadership challenges—and whose ability matches their interest—are the best candidates for senior leadership positions in the hospital and leadership roles on the health system board. Over time the group will come to lead the system, replicating the model of the revered group practices identified in Chapter 5. This approach is exemplified in the quote of one system CEO who noted: "Today most hospitals employ physicians to fill beds and meet facility needs. Our strategic goal is to transform into a physician-directed health system where the hospital is simply one of many tools the physicians use to organize and deliver superb care for our community" (Rick Pearce, CEO and

President, Riverside Health System, Newport News, VA; personal communication).

BRANDING AN INTEGRATED SYSTEM

This chapter has advocated that a hospital engage in careful even-handedness in terms of marketing the services and skills of medical staff physicians as a strategy to mitigate tension between its group practice members and independent physicians. As the balance of group and independent physicians shifts, and dependence on independent physicians wanes, the need for such a strategy diminishes, allowing the health system to differentiate itself in the marketplace by advertising how tight integration with its own physician group allows for more patient-friendly, efficient, high-quality, cost-effective care. This message will attract increasing numbers of discerning patients and payers.

CONCLUSION

Hospitals that simply employ physicians do not create a new delivery model to meet twenty-first-century expectations. Health systems that create owned or affiliated practice groups have greater potential to create a truly integrated enterprise. Organizations that invest heavily in developing the physician leadership of these groups have the greatest potential to create innovative and successful new care delivery models. To accomplish this aim, these organizations will have to cede greater levels of control over health system affairs to their emerging group and its cadre of physician leaders. In the future, we can expect to see greater numbers of hospital CEOs who are physicians, governing boards chaired by doctors, and senior health system management positions held by individuals with medical degrees. The hospital affiliated group practice will be an increasingly important place to forge such future leaders for the country's healthcare systems.

Conclusion

Momentum for health reform is reaching an all-time high as this book goes to press. Change is in the air, but so is resistance and vast uncertainty. What will healthcare delivery in the United States look like 20 years from now? This question is difficult to answer, but we can safely say that it will be radically different from today's model. The United States cannot sustain cost increases at the current trajectory, nor will those who pay for insured care be willing to settle for what currently are mixed results in terms of quality and safety. In addition, the passage of time will take its inevitable toll on the current generation of healthcare leaders, and many will retire. The pace of clinical innovation suggests that routine treatment methodologies of the future will resemble those described in today's science fiction. Under these inexorable pressures, the current system of payment and care delivery will be overtaken at some point by a wave of radical, discontinuous change.

On the other hand, some aspects of healthcare delivery will not change at all. The plea for quality, safety, and value will not disappear, and the sick will continue to hope for individualized, personalized care that combines high tech and high touch. Practitioners will continue to want work that is personally rewarding and adequately remunerated. Patient-centered integration of care across sites and types of service will become even more critical to satisfying these longstanding demands.

To prepare for the uncertainty of the future, healthcare institutions must build approaches to care delivery that involve physicians in the search for solutions, link ambulatory and inpatient care, embrace change, and commit to innovation. The development of hospital affiliated group practices paves a path toward these goals. These practices will anchor and direct the integrated approach to care delivery envisioned by today's healthcare futurists. Practice leaders will be able to achieve the elusive goal of moderating costs while delivering great care.

The values that define America's leading group practices, and their ability to innovate care delivery by combining physician involvement with executive skills, are a model for every hospital and health system. For institutions starting down this road, how quickly can this model be achieved? The answer depends on the wide range of factors discussed in this book. How committed are the health system's leaders? What resources can be allocated for this initiative? Is the physician community receptive to the idea, or will interest need to be cultivated? How does hospital location affect recruitment and regional competition? Regardless of local circumstances, most health systems seriously committed to the path we have outlined should be able to develop a fully functioning group practice within five years. This time frame may seem short, but time is of the essence. Group formation should begin now, not at the end of this wave of change.

Consumers are easily chagrined—and sometimes mortified—by the haphazard nature of healthcare delivery across the United States today. The authors of this book are optimistic that American ingenuity; the longstanding values of professional medicine; and the collaboration of thoughtful physicians, hospital administrators, board members, politicians, payers, and policy experts can combine to build fully integrated care delivery systems—the wellsprings of a better future.

References

American Board of Internal Medicine (ABIM) Foundation. 2009. "Medical Professionalism in the New Millennium: A Physician Charter." [Online information; retrieved 3/4/09.] www.abimfoundation.org/professionalism/charter.shtm.

Argyris, C. 1960. *Understanding Organizational Behavior.* Homewood, IL: Dorsey Press.

Atchison, T., and J. Bujak. 2001. *Leading Transformational Change: The Physician–Executive Partnership.* Chicago: Health Administration Press.

Beery, L., and K. Seltman. 2008. *Management Lessons from Mayo Clinic: Inside One of the World's Most Admired Service Organizations.* New York: McGraw-Hill.

Berwick, D. M., T. W. Nolan, and J. Whittington. 2008. "The Triple Aim: Care, Health, and Cost." *Health Affairs* 27 (3): 759–69.

Bujak, J. 2008. *Inside the Physician Mind: Finding Common Ground with Doctors.* Chicago: Health Administration Press.

Collins, J. 2001. *Good to Great: Why Some Companies Make the Leap...And Others Don't.* New York: Harper Collins.

Community Care of North Carolina. 2008. "Program Overview." [Online information; retrieved 6/24/08.] www.communitycarenc.com.

Croasdale, M. 2006. "AAMC Seeks 30% Hike in Enrollment." [Online article; retrieved 6/5/09.] www.ama-assn.org/amednews/2006/07/10/prsd0710.htm.

Diamond, M. A. 2003. "Organizational Immersion and Diagnosis: The Work of Harry Levinson." *Organisational and Social Dynamics: An International Journal for the Integration of Psychoanalytic, Systemic and Group Relations Perspectives* 3 (2): 1–18.

Institute of Medicine (IOM). 2001. *Crossing the Quality Chasm: A New Health System for the 21st Century.* Washington, DC: National Academies Press.

———. 2000. *To Err Is Human: Building a Safer Health System.* Washington, DC: National Academies Press.

Kaplan, R., and D. Norton. 1996. *The Balanced Scorecard: Translating Strategy into Action.* Boston: Harvard Business School Press.

Lister, E. D. 1998. "I Can't Believe They Think I'd…." *Physician Executive* 24 (4): 24–25, 28.

Merritt Hawkins & Associates. 2008. "The Physicians' Perspective: Medical Practice in 2008." [Online information; retrieved 6/5/09.] www.physiciansfoundations.org/usr_doc/PF_Survey_Report.pdf.

Rittenhouse, D. R., L. P. Casalino, R. R. Gillies, S. M. Shortell, and B. Lau. 2008. "Measuring the Medical Home Infrastructure in Large Medical Groups." *Health Affairs* 27 (5): 1246–58.

Silversin, J., and M. J. Kornacki. 2000. *Leading Physicians Through Change: How to Achieve and Sustain Results.* Tampa, FL: American College of Physician Executives.

State of North Carolina, Office of the Governor. 2007. "Gov. Easley Announces Community Care Saves Taxpayers $231 Million." Press release, September 25. [Online information; retrieved 6/24/08.] www.communitycarenc.com/PDFDocs/InnovPress.pdf.

Sterns, J. B. 2007. "Quality, Efficiency, and Organizational Structure." *Journal of Health Care Finance* 34 (1): 100–07.

U.S. Department of Health and Human Services. 2006. "Physician Supply and Demand: Projections to 2020." [Online information; retrieved 6/5/09.] http://bhpr.hrsa.gov/healthworkforce/reports/physiciansupply demand/currentphysicianwork force.htm.

Index

Academic institutions, liaisons with group practices, 171–172

Accountability: in decision making, 63; for group practice development, 79; of group practice members, 71, 122, 176; of medical directors, 86, 111; of office staff members, 142; of physician leaders, 118–119

Accreditation, 182–183

Accreditation Association for Ambulatory Health Care, 183

Administrator-physician relationship, 5; collaboration in, 119; effect of managed care on, 6–7

Administrators: attitudes toward physician leaders, 78; commitment to group practices, 77–80; as group practice managers, 69–70, 94; interaction with medical directors, 111, 113; physicians' distrust toward, 21, 63; with practice management

experience, 49; supportive of group practices, 77–79

Agency for Healthcare Research and Quality (AHRQ), 134–135

Ambassadorship function, of group practice boards, 94–95, 96–97

Ambulatory care. *See also* Outpatient care facilities; Outpatient care practices: hospitals' management of, 49; implication for hospital-physician relations, 7, 10–11; provided by specialists, 7; standardization of, 51–52

Ambulatory care facilities: physicians' ownership of, 37–38; surgery centers, 14

American Association for Accreditation of Ambulatory Surgery Facilities, 183

American Board of Internal Medicine, Medicaid Professional

into group practices, 201–202

Clinical pathways, 9

Co-branding, 25

Codes, of professional conduct, 9, 133, 188

Coding, 49, 156–157

Collaboration: administrator–medical director, 111; administrator–physician, 119; among group practice members, 51, 64, 65, 123, 202; commitment to, 131; hospital–physician, 8, 11, 22, 23, 45–46; manager–physician, 80; physician leaders' skills in, 79

Collegiality, 122

Colocation, of group practice physicians, 68, 125

Commitment: of group practice members, 121; in hospital-physician relationship, 24; institutional, to group practices, 77–81; personal, 20; as physician covenant component, 130–132; professional, 22–23

Commonwealth Fund, 66–67

Communication, 19–21, 97

Compacts. *See also* Covenants: physician–hospital, 36–37

Compensation, 71, 74, 125, 152, 154–156. *See also* Income; Reimbursement; Revenue: for call services, 36–37; for creativity and initiative, 147; discretionary dimension of, 155; for dual employment, 189–190; for emergency room coverage, 36–37; excessive, 184–185;

from for-profit organizations, 184; for group practice board members, 102; guidelines for, 154–156; as incentive, 127; legal and regulatory issues affecting, 183–187; productivity-based, 127, 151, 154–155, 156; relative value unit-based, 147, 150, 154; from tax-exempt organizations, 184–185

Compensation committees, 82–83, 89

Compensation consultants, 152, 154

Competition: federal government's support for, 195; hospital–physician, 7–8, 10–11, 40; physicians' attitudes toward, 203

Computerized provider entry systems (CPOE), 9

Concierge medicine, 46

Conduct, codes of, 9, 133, 188

Confidentiality, 97, 99, 133, 168, 190

Conflict, group practice boards' avoidance of, 99

Conflict of interest, 187–188, 206–207

Conflict resolution, 71, 132

Contracts: at-risk, 116; corporate practice of medicine restrictions and, 180; "co-terminus" provisions of, 169; employment, 19, 26, 48–49, 115, 193–194; exclusive, 26, 193–194, 207–208; with payers, negotiation of, 49, 50; performance

35–36

Economic alignment, hospital–physician, 24–25
Economic model, of group practice, 147–150
Effectiveness, 83–84
Efficiency, 59–60, 83–84, 141, 158–159
Electronic medical record (EMR) systems, 24–25; cost of implementation of, 34, 67–68; purchase of, 149; use by group practices, 64, 65, 145, 170, 172, 173; use by hospital-employed physicians, 51; use in practice profiling, 172, 173; younger physicians' preference for, 35
Emergency room physicians, 36–37, 201, 202
Employment relationships. *See also* Hospital employment, of physicians: younger physicians' preference for, 35–36
Empowerment, 122, 176
Endoscopic procedures, outpatient, 14
Entrepreneurship, of physicians, 35
Errors, preventable, 41
Evidence-based medicine, 170–171
Executives, of healthcare systems. *See also* Chief executive officers (CEOs); Chief medical officers (CMOs); Physician executives: commitment to group practice

formation, 77–80
Expectations: about group practice formation, 83; about group practice profitability, 147–150; about hospital-employed physicians, 54–55; of group practice members, 176

Federal Trade Commission (FTC), 195
Finance directors, 88
Financial issues, in group practice formation, 67–68
Foundation Model, 182
Fraud, in coding, 156

Gainsharing, 27–28, 151–152
Geisinger Health System, 61, 66
Goals, relationship to oversight, 96
Goal setting, by group practice boards, 96
Good to Great (Collins), 23
Goodwill, 34, 41, 43n, 47, 148, 194
Governance: differentiated from management, 94; of hospital group practices. *See* Hospital group practice boards
Group practices. *See* Hospital group practices
Guidance, 94–95

Harvard Business School, 96
Havens, L. L., 158
Healthcare: patient-centered, 122, 131, 134, 139; physician-centered, 63, 122

Healthcare costs, inflation of, 5

Healthcare delivery: future of, 211–212; integrated systems for, 65–67; variations in, 167–168

Healthcare Facilities Accreditation Program, 182

Healthcare Financial Management Association, 156

Healthcare system: improvement of, ix; physician-directed, 208; reform of, 211

Health Systems Law Institute, 178

Hospital(s). *See also* Inpatient care; *names of specific hospitals:* community, 4, 7, 8; corporate management of, 6; for-profit, 6, 184; leadership of, 204–206; lengths-of-stay in, 4; not-for-profit, 6, 184; physician development plans of, 13–14; specialty, 8, 10–11

Hospital affiliations, of physicians. *See also* Hospital employment, of physicians: expansion of, 5; insurance companies' requirements for, 14–15; prestige associated with, 3–4; of primary care physicians, 14–15

Hospital boards: conflict of interest policies of, 187, 188; group practice development evaluations by, 67–71; Internal Revenue Service rules regarding, 180, 181; physician members, 180–181, 206–207; supportive of group practices, 79

Hospital employment, of physicians, 25–28; advantages of, 25–26; allocation of cost and income in, 50; as dual employment, 187–188; gainsharing-based, 27–28; group practice exclusion and, 126–127; *versus* hospital practice acquisition, 41–42; hospitals' emerging interest in, 36–41; motivations for, 33–36, 127; physicians' preferences in, 45–46; short-term, 42; without integrated group practices, 59–61

Hospital group practice(s): advantages of, 61–67; alignment with independent practices, 202–203; ancillary revenue from, 148–149, 151; assimilation of hospital-based services into, 201–202; basic skills needed for, 45–55; bylaws of, 192; conflict with medical staff, 163–164; conflict with private practice physicians, 94; early stages of, 126–128; financial resources of, 67–68; formation of, 46–47, 67–71, 126–128; guiding principles of, 91–92; healthcare leadership role of, 208–209; implementation of, 72–74; informing the public about, 81; institutional commitment to, 77–79; integrated healthcare approach of, 65–67, 209, 212; legal and regulatory issues affecting, 177–197; measures of success of, 71–72; multispecialty, 202; as "one-stop shopping," 142; opposition to, 62, 77–81; participation in hospital/health system governance, 206–207; participation in hospital leadership, 204–206; policies and procedures of, 192; restrictive bylaws affecting, 206; single-specialty, 26, 180, 202; successful, 61–65; value structure of, 62–63

Hospital group practice boards, 71, 91–103; authority of, 92–93; bylaws of, 192; chairperson's role in, 101–102; compensation for, 102; composition and committee structure of, 82–84, 89, 99–100, 101; differentiated from medical staff, 93–94; election of members, 88; formal, induction of, 88; functions and responsibilities of, 91–92, 94–98; governance education for, 101; governance principles of, 99; interim, 81–84, 88, 89; learning process within, 100–101; legal duties of, 98–99; medical director members of, 94, 101, 102; members' differences of opinion, 99; membership criteria for, 93–94; oversight of medical directors by, 86; practice administrator members of, 94, 101; relationships with hospitals/health systems, 91–93; role of, 84–85; self-regulation of, 97–98

Hospitalists, 14; exclusive contracts with, 26; as group practice members, 201; "shift work" approach of, 202

Hospital–physician alignment/relationship, 3–12; adversarial nature of, 5–7; competition in, 7–8, 10–11; contractual relationships for, 28, 29–30; creation of, 18–31; diagnosis-related groups and, 5–6; distrust in, 53; economic incentive alignment in, 4; economic options for, 24–25; "golden age" of, 5; independent physicians' involvement in, 202–203; medical specialization and, 4; medical technology and, 4; outpatient practice and, 7–8, 10; practice culture and, 63–64; as professional community, 4–5; statutory barriers to, 8; strategies for, 13–31; during twentieth century, 3–7; into the during twenty-first century, 7–11

Hulefeld, Mike, 113

Incident review, 117, 157

Income: expectations regarding, 150; of hospital-employed physicians, 49, 50

Incompetency, of group practice members, 169

Incorporation, of physician practices, 182

Independent practice physicians, 46; hospitals' alignment with, 202–203; marketing assistance for, 144–145; as medical directors, 204; opposition to group practices, 144, 206, 209

Industry–physician relationships, 188

Inflation, of medical costs, 5

Information technology, 51, 64, 145. *See also* Electronic medical record (EMR) systems

Infrastructure: for credentialing and privileging, 164–166; for group practices, 50–51, 71, 141–144; for hospital-employed physicians, 60–61; hospitals' provision of, 25–26; importance of, 139; for organized medical staffs, 206

Innovation, within group practices, 65, 122–123

Inpatient care, provided by specialists, 7

Institute of Medicine, *Crossing the Quality Chasm*, 75

Intended practice plans, 24

Internal Revenue Service (IRS), 179, 180, 184–185

Inurement, private, 184–185, 189, 194

Investments, strategic differentiated from operational, 149

Joint Commission, The, 182

Joint ventures, 11, 26–27, 180

Journal of Health Care Finance, 167

Lawyers, involvement in group practice formation, 177–178

Leadership. *See also* Physician leaders; Physician leadership: of hospitals, 204–206

Leaves of absence, 8, 38–39

Legal issues, affecting group practices, 177–197; accreditation, 182–183; checklist for, 196; compensation, 183–185; corporate practice of medicine, 180, 181–182; corporate relationships, 178–181; counsel for group practices, 177–178; recruitment of physicians, 192–194

Levinson, Harry, 130

Liaison role, of physician executives, 60

Lifestyle choices, of physicians, 8–9, 11, 35, 38, 135

Location, of group practice offices, 68, 125, 149

Loyalty, 4, 6, 7, 99, 142

Malpractice liability, 8, 157, 158, 164

Managed care, 6–7, 37

Management: differentiated from governance, 94; physicians' involvement in, 4

Managers: adversarial relationships with physicians, 7; commitment to group practices, 77–78, 80–81; physicians as, 209; supportive of group practices, 77–79

Marketing: co-branding and, 25; of group practices, 52–53; of independent practices,

144–145; of medical staff's services, 209

Mayo Clinic, 61–62, 65

Medicaid, 4, 182

Medicaid patients, 149–150

Medical directors: accountability of, 86; of clinical services and programs, 204; credibility of, 111, 113; with group practice management experience, 85–86; of group practices, 85–86, 94, 110–118; incumbent, 86–87; interaction with administrators, 111, 113; as leaders, 107, 204; "managed care," 116; part-time, 118; priorities of, 119; recruitment and development of, 85–86, 89, 109–111, 204; reporting relations of, 86, 111, 112; roles and responsibilities of, 108, 111–118; skills and competencies of, 110–111

Medical education, 39

Medical Group Management Association, 156, 192

Medical homes, 66–67, 151–152

Medical records, computerization of. *See* Electronic medical record (EMR) systems

Medical school graduates, 39

Medical school students, female, 8

Medical staff: closed *versus* open, 207–208; differentiated from physician practice community, 14–15; expansion of, 5; group practice physicians employed as, 189–190; involvement in peer review, 168; opposition to group practice, 163–164; organized, 4, 205–206

Medical staff development plans, 13–14, 15–17

Medical staff executive committees, 41, 94, 109

Medical technology, 4, 207

Medicare: Conditions of Participation, 182, 205; effect on hospital–physician relations, 4; physician payment schedule of, 34, 151–152; residency position funding by, 39

Medicare patients, 149–150

Medicare Payment Advisory Commission, 151–152

Meetings, 19, 20, 80–81

Mentoring: of group practice board members, 101–102; of group practice medical directors, 110; of group practice physicians, 114, 124; of hospital-employed physicians, 48; of physician leaders, 53–54, 85, 108, 119

Micromanagement, 96

Misconduct, disciplining process for, 132, 133–134

Mission, of group practice board members, 98

Mission statements, 91–92, 95, 130

Motivation, 33–36, 107–108, 127–128

Multidisciplinary physician groups. *See* Hospital group practices

National Committee for Quality Assurance, 66, 183
National Patient Safety Foundation, 134
National Practitioner Data Bank, 163, 164, 169, 176n
Negligence, 8
Negotiation, of contracts, 49, 50
"Never" events, 41
Norton, David, 96

Ochsner Clinic, 61, 62
Ochsner Health System, 62
Ochsner Medical Center, 111, 113
Office design, 125, 146
Office managers, 52
Office of Inspector General (OIG), 28, 186, 191
Office space, 68, 141–142
Office staff, 52, 87–88, 141, 142–144, 146, 147
Open heart surgery, "warranties" for, 66
Operating councils, 19, 204–205
Operational guidelines, 92
Operations committees, 83–84, 89
Outpatient care facilities, physicians' investments in, 7–8
Outpatient care practices: effect of managed care on, 37; hospital–patient relations and, 7–8, 10; increase in, 37–38; of specialists, 15
Outreach: by group practice boards, 94–95, 96–97; as hospital–physician alignment strategy, 20; to independent practice physicians, 203

Overhead, "direct," 155
Oversight, by group practice boards, 94–95, 96
Ownership: of ambulatory care facilities, 37–38; of group practices, 179; of hospitals, 4

Palo Alto Foundation Medical Group, 143, 174
Part-time employment, of physicians, 8, 35, 43n
Patient access, to group practice physicians, 117
Patient-centered healthcare, 122, 131, 134, 149
Patient-centered medical homes (PCMHs), 66–67, 151–152
Patient safety goals, 9
Patient satisfaction, 18, 65, 116, 202
Pay-for-performance reimbursement, 10, 40–41, 151; formulas for, 8; gainsharing in, 28; goals for, 40–41; integrated approach to, 151, 153–154; quality outcomes-based, 116; regulatory issues regarding, 186; safety outcomes-based, 116
Peer review process, 11, 20–22, 64, 94, 166–167, 168, 176, 206
Performance: contractual provisions for, 189–190; core measures for, 9; expectations about, 47; problematic, 169; transparency regarding, 8, 11

Performance evaluation and review, 55, 96, 124, 143–144

Performance improvement, 176

Personnel management, 47, 87, 113–118, 134

Physician(s). See also Independent practice physicians; Physician leaders; Physician executives; Primary care physicians; Private practice physicians; Specialists: community, 70; demographics of, 8; older, 35; part-time administrative activities of, 155; shortage of, 14, 37–40; younger, 35–36, 38, 135

Physician development plans, 13–14

Physician executives: dual clinician-administrative role of, 111, 113; rise of, 106–107; skills and competencies of, 107–108

Physician–hospital compacts, 36–37

Physician leaders, 48; administrators' attitudes toward, 78; beliefs and behaviors affecting, 105–106; clinical practice involvement of, 53, 54; credibility of, 54; development of, 114, 118–119; educational opportunities for, 106–107; of group practices, 70, 105–120, 135–136; influence on group cohesiveness, 135–136; as medical directors, 107, 204; mentoring of, 53–54, 85, 108, 119; as operating council members, 205; roles and responsibilities

of, 53–54, 55; skills and competencies of, 79, 107–108

Physician leadership: of academic institutions, 106; curriculum in, 108; decentralization of, 118–119; group-focused *versus* hospital-focused, 109; group practice boards' role in, 92–93; of group practices, 53–54; for hospital–physician alignment, 21–22; of hospitals/healthcare systems, 208–209; necessity for, 106

Physician practice community, 14–15, 15–17

Physician practices: assets of, 47, 148; decentralization of, 7; hospitals' acquisition of, 5–6, 11, 41–32, 46–47, 193–194. See also Hospital group practices; incorporation of, 182; market value of, 47; purchasing arrangements for, 148

Physicians and Physician Organizations Law Institute, 178

Physician executives, 60, 84–87

Practice culture. See Culture, of group practice

Practice environment, 50–51

Practice management, 146–147

Practice management companies, 6

Practice management skills, 51–53

Practice management teams, 87–88, 142

Practice managers, 72–73,

143–144

Practice profiling, 172, 173

Practice quality committees, 168–169

Pricing, value-based, 41

Primary care physicians, 14; as group practice members, 201; as specialist referral source, 67–68, 174; specialists' assistance to, 174

Private practice, operational complexity of, 33–34

Private practice physicians, 7; conflict with group practices, 94; constraints on, 33–34; employed as hospital staff, 69; income of, 38; office expenses of, 33–34; shortage of, 38; as specialist referral source, 67–68

Privileging process, 161–166

Problem-solving skills, 133

Process design, 125

Process improvement, 117–118, 125–126, 159

Productivity, 38–39, 41–42, 122; as basis for compensation, 127, 151, 154–155, 156; expectations regarding, 54–55; hospitals' expectations regarding, 47; monitoring of, 115–116; relative value unit-based calculation of, 154

Professional affairs committees, 114

Professional development, 114

Professionalism, 9, 10, 22–23

Professional life, constraints of private practice on, 34–35

Professional services agreements (PSA), 182

Profiling, of group practices, 172, 173

Profitability, of group practices, 147–150

Prospective payment systems, 5

Protocol development, 170–172

Quality, effect of practice culture on, 134–135

Quality committees, 83, 89, 170

Quality goals, 116–117

Quality improvement, 125–126, 167–169

Rapid cycle improvement, 158–159

Recruitment, of physicians, 13–14, 39–40, 42, 48–49, 69, 123; guidelines for, 128–129; implication for practice culture, 128–130; legal and regulatory issues affecting, 192–194; of medical directors, 85–86, 89, 109–110; medical director's role in, 114; plans and strategies for, 15–16, 23–24, 114

Recruitment committees, 129–130

Referral leakage, 174

Referrals: anti-kickback laws regarding, 8, 10, 177, 186, 189, 194; to group practice members, 71; from group practice physicians, 45; from hospital-affiliated physicians, 203; from independent practice physicians, 203; to independent practice physicians, 203; medical staff applicants and, 24; to non–group practice members, 174, 175; physicians' control of, 7–8; from primary care physicians, 67–68, 174; from private practice physicians, 67–68; tracking patterns of, 174–175

Regulatory issues: accreditation, 182–183; affecting hospital group practices, 177–197; affecting hospitals' medical staffs, 4; affecting hospital–physician relations, 8, 11; checklist for, 196; compensation, 183–187; corporate compliance activities, 190–191; corporate practice of medicine, 180, 181–182; recruitment of physicians, 192–194

Reimbursement. *See also specific types of reimbursement:* constraints on, 34; cost-based, 4; diagnosis-related group-based, 5; "global case," 152; integrated approach in, 152, 153; for Medicare and Medicaid patients, 149–150; trends in, 151–152

Relative value units (RVUs), 147, 150, 154, 173

Remediation, in hospital–physician relations, 48

Research, 171–172, 188

Responsiveness, in hospital–physician relations, 20–21

Retention, of physicians, 23–24, 48

Retirement, 35, 39, 42–43n, 211

Return on investment (ROI), 148, 149

Revenue: from ancillary services, 148–149, 151; expected, as basis for budgets, 151; from hospital-employed physicians, 50

Risk management, 117, 157–158, 167

Rituals, 135–136

Riverside Medical Group Physician Covenant, 131

Robinson-Patman Act, 195

Role modeling, 124

Safety issues, 116–117, 134–135

Scott & White Clinic, 98, 158

Self-governance, of group practices, 70, 71. *See also* Hospital group practice boards

Self-regulation, of group practice boards, 97–98

Service(s): high-acuity, 208; as hospital–physician alignment strategy, 18–19, 25; non-group providers of, 207–208; to patients, 117; as professional value, 22

Sherman Act, 195

"Shift work" approach, 202

Six Sigma, 159

Specialists. *See also* Referrals: exclusive contracts with, 26; as group practice members, 201; hospital-based, 201–202; income of, 38; inpatient care provided by, 7, 38; interaction with primary care physicians,

174; outpatient care provided by, 7, 15, 38

Specialties, medical, 4

Standardization: of ambulatory care practices, 51–52; of clinical protocol, 170; of office practice, 146–147, 159

Stark laws, 8, 11, 24–26, 185–186, 193

Strategic analysis, in medical staff development planning, 16–17

Strategic planning: for group practice development, 72, 77–89, 139–141; for hospital–physician alignment, 13–31

Structural relationships, group practices/health systems, 178–181

Subsidiary corporations, 178–179

Supervision, of physician leaders, 108, 119

Tax Equity and Fiscal Responsibility Act (TEFRA), 5

Tax-exempt status, 179, 183–185

Teamwork, in group practice, 64, 65

Termination, of employment: of group practice members, 114, 169; of hospital-employed physicians, 189–190; of medical staff, 169, 189–190

Third-party payers, transparency demands from, 8

Toyota, Lean production system of, 159

Transparency: of compensation plans, 154; of group practice

boards' decision making, 97; of medical directors' appointment process, 204; regarding hospital/physician performance, 8, 11

Uninsured patients, 7–8, 149–150

URAC (Utilization Review Accreditation Commission), 183

Utilization departments, 5–6

Utilization management and review, 116, 167–168

Values: of group practices, 123; of integrated care delivery systems, 167; professional, 22–23, 134

Value shifts, among younger physicians, 35–36

Value statements, 91–92, 95, 130

Vice president for medical affairs (VPMA), 21–22, 85, 86, 106–107, 109, 204

Vision statements, 91–92, 95, 130

Volunteer services, of physicians, 36

"Warranties," for open heart surgery, 66

Wellness committees, 114

Women, as physicians, 8, 38–39

Work hours, of physicians, 8, 20, 38–39

About the Authors

Eric Lister, MD, is a physician and consultant to healthcare organizations. He works throughout the healthcare industry—with group practices, hospitals, insurers, professional societies, manufacturers, and large integrated systems.

Dr. Lister has published a wide variety of articles addressing healthcare governance, the consultation process, group practice leadership, and the development of organizational cohesion. He has served as a faculty member for the American College of Physician Executives, the New England Healthcare Assembly, the Group Practice Improvement Network, the Governance Institute, the American Hospital Association's Center for Healthcare Governance, and the American Medical Group Association. He lectures widely on topics related to governance, quality, leadership, and the relationship between America's physicians and hospitals.

In 2002, he was selected by the Massachusetts Hospital Association to co-direct the Healthcare Trustee Institute, a regional resource for trustee education. From 2002 to 2004, he worked with the National Quality Forum (NQF) on the creation of NQF's landmark document, *Hospital Governing Boards and Quality of Care: A Call to Responsibility*. In 2007, he was asked by the Leapfrog Group to be one of two course directors of its 2008 conference, "The Future of Hospital Governance: Quality at the Leading Edge."

Initially trained as a psychiatrist at Duke University and Harvard, Dr. Lister taught at Harvard and Tufts Medical Schools, served as the medical director of a 65-bed psychiatric hospital, and was a founding partner of a large group mental health practice before moving from clinical practice to full-time consulting work in 2000.

Dr. Lister and his wife are the proud parents of two grown daughters. When not at work, Dr. Lister enjoys kayaking and woodworking.

Todd Sagin, MD, JD, is a physician executive recognized across the nation for his work with hospital boards, medical staffs, and physician organizations. He is a cofounder of HG Healthcare Consultants, LLC, which provides guidance on a wide range of healthcare issues. He previously served for over half a decade as the vice president and national medical director of The Greeley Company, a division of HCPro, Inc. Dr. Sagin is frequently asked to assist hospitals and physicians in developing strong working relationships amid increasing competition and diverging interests. Over the past decade, he has worked with several hundred of the nation's medical staffs on issues ranging from organizational redesign and bylaw revision to medical staff strategic planning, peer review effectiveness, credentialing, and leadership development. In recent years, he has assisted numerous health systems develop owned or affiliated multidisciplinary group practices.

Dr. Sagin is a popular public speaker. He won the Golden Apple teaching award at Temple University School of Medicine, where he was vice president and chief medical officer of the university's health system. He frequently facilitates board and medical staff retreats and delivers leadership education to trustees and physician leaders. Dr. Sagin is a regular faculty member of The Governance Institute and a principal advisor and lecturer for its Medical Leadership Institute. He is board certified in family medicine and currently practices at Community Volunteers in Medicine in West Chester, PA.